Yoga - Exploring the Health Benefits and Diverse Dimensions

Edited by Rameswar Pal

Published in London, United Kingdom

Yoga - Exploring the Health Benefits and Diverse Dimensions
http://dx.doi.org/10.5772/intechopen.1000297
Edited by Rameswar Pal

Contributors
Deepshikha Thakur, Fadi Kayale, Hin Hung Sik, Holly Pollard-Wright, Junling Gao, Rameswar Pal, Sarah Green, Sobika Rao, Stephen Parker

First published in London, United Kingdom, 2024 by IntechOpen
IntechOpen is the global imprint of INTECHOPEN LIMITED, registered in England and Wales, registration number: 11086078, 167-169 Great Portland Street, London, W1W 5PF, United Kingdom

British Library Cataloguing-in-Publication Data
A catalogue record for this book is available from the British Library

Additional hard and PDF copies can be obtained from orders@intechopen.com

Yoga - Exploring the Health Benefits and Diverse Dimensions
Edited by Rameswar Pal
p. cm.
Print ISBN 978-0-85466-005-6
Online ISBN 978-0-85466-004-9
eBook (PDF) ISBN 978-0-85466-006-3

[19] ICOLD. Use of granular filters and drains in embankment dams. Bulletin 95; 1994

[20] Sherard JL, Dunnigan LJ. Critical filters for impervious soils. Journal of Geotechnical Engineering. 1989;**115**(7):927-947

[21] USACE. Appendix D–Filter Design. EM 1110-2-1913; 2000

[22] USBR. Protective filters. Design standards No. 13 – Embankment dams, chap 5; 2000

[23] USSCS. Gradation design of sand and gravel filters. Chapter 26. In: Part 633 National Engineering Handbook. United States Department of Agriculture; 1994

[24] Sherard JL, Woodward RJ, Gizinski SF, Clvenger WA. Earth and earth rock dams. New York: Wiley; 1967

[25] López-Acosta NP. Modelado numérico de problemas de flujo de agua. Memorias de la XXVII Reunión Nacional de Ingeniería Geotécnica. Puerto Vallarta, Jalisco, México: Sociedad Mexicana de Ingeniería Geotécnica (SMIG); 2014

[26] López-Acosta NP, González JL. Study of water flow in dams using successive overrelaxations. Water Technology and Sciences. 2015:43-58 (in Spanish)

[27] López-Acosta NP, Promotor JA. Flujo de agua en suelos parcialmente saturados y su aplicación a la ingeniería geotécnica. In: Serie de Investigación y Desarrollo. México, DF, México: Instituto de Ingeniería - UNAM; 2016

[28] López-Acosta NP, De la Fuente H, Auvinet G. Safety of a protection levee under rapid drawdown conditions. Coupled analysis of transient seepage and stability. In: Proceedings of the 18th International Conference on Soil Mechanics and Geotechnical Engineering; Technical Committe 210+201 (Dykes, Leeves and Dams); Paris, France. 2013. pp. 3305-3308

[29] López-Acosta NP. Flujo de agua en suelos. Capítulo 9 del Manual de Diseño de Obras Civiles [Sección B. Geotecnia. Tema 2. Mecánica de Suelos]. México: Comisión Federal de Electricidad; 2016

[30] González JL, López-Acosta NP. Application of the successive overrelaxation technique to confined and unconfined water flow problems (In Spanish). XXVII Reunión Nacional de Ingeneiría Geotécnica. Puerto Vallarta, Jalisco, MEX: Sociedad Mexicana de Ingeniería Geotécnica; 2014. p. 10

[31] Arreguín FI, Murillo R, Marengo H. Inventario Nacional de Presas. Tecnología y Ciencias Del Agua. 2013;**4**(4):179-185

[32] Cooper B. Dam safety management within a risk framework, an Australian dam safety regulator´s perspective. In: 81st Annual Meeting of the International Commission on Large Dams; 2013

For EU product safety concerns:
IN TECH d.o.o., Prolaz Marije Krucifikse Kozulić 3, 51000 Rijeka, Croatia,
info@intechopen.com or visit our website at intechopen.com.

Meet the editor

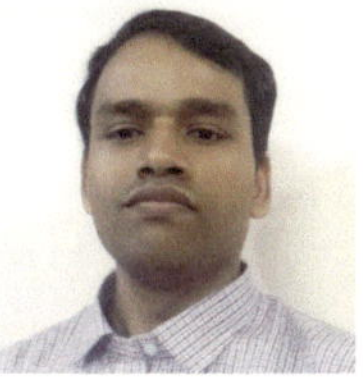

Dr. Rameswar Pal is an Assistant Professor of Human Physiology at Morarji Desai National Institute of Yoga, Ministry of Ayush, Government of India. He was awarded a Ph.D. in Life Sciences from Bharathiar University, India. He completed his Ph.D. thesis work at the Defence Institute of Physiology & Allied Sciences (DIPAS), Defence Research & Development Organisation (DRDO), Ministry of Defence, Government of India. He is a life member of the Association of Physiologists and Pharmacologists of India (APPI), the Physiological Society of India (PSI), and the Indian Science Congress Association (ISCA). He has published a book chapter and many full papers. He has also published several abstracts in conference proceedings and delivered many lectures. He has been awarded a travel grant to attend the 1st Tehran IBRO/APRC Associate School of Cognitive Neurosciences on Functional Human Brain Mapping in Tehran, Iran, in 2015. He was also awarded "The Sushila Thaker Prakriti Mandir Prize" for research investigation in Natural Health, Naturopathy, and Yoga by the APPI at APPICON 2015.

Contents

Preface

Yoga is an Indian traditional heritage. It is based on the Sanskrit word yuj, which means "to join." In spiritual terms, yoga is about connecting the individual to the whole. Practically, it brings your body, mind, and emotions into harmony.

There are several distinct branches of yoga, each of which has been extensively explained in various texts. These branches include Raja yoga, Hatha yoga, Jnana yoga, Karma yoga, Bhakti yoga, Mantra yoga, Kundalini yoga, and Laya yoga.

Yoga – Exploring the Health Benefits and Diverse Dimensions explores different dimensions of yoga, such as traditional knowledge, health impacts, and other aspects. It also provides insight into Patanjali's Chitta Prasadamnam for mental well-being, the health impacts of different components of yoga (such as asana pranayama yoga Nidra), and yoga rehabilitation therapy. Yoga is a very vast field of research, making it impossible to cover all aspects in a single book. However, we address many related topics in this volume.

Dr. Rameswar Pal
Department of Human Physiology,
Morarji Desai National Institute of Yoga,
Ministry of Ayush,
Government of India,
New Delhi, India

Chapter 1

Importance of Patanjali's Chitta Prasadanam for Mental Wellbeing

Deepshikha Thakur

Abstract

The mind has a built-in propensity to be drawn to the outside environment. The ability to gaze within is not inherent in the mind. Therefore, challenges present themselves when attempting to focus inward. However, these barriers are not distinct from consciousness; rather, they are a component of it. They are inevitable and have specific points in the framework of consciousness. Such contaminants and impediments must first be eliminated. The mind must be cleared, and inner calm must be brought about to be able to focus. The Patanjali Yoga Sutra 1.33 refers to "Chitta Prasadanam," which literally translates as Calm mind. "Maitri Karuna Muditopekshanam" is how it is spelt. "Bhavnatas Chitta Prasadanam Sukh Dukh Punya Apunya Vishyanayam." According to the Sutra, your mind is guided toward tranquility and peace when you have a favorable attitude toward both happy and unhappy individuals, are only affected by virtues, and do not even consider the drawbacks.

Keywords: chitta, chitta prasadanam, panch klesha, Yogantraya, mental health

1. Introduction

Afflictions (anything that produces pain or suffering) are the primary cause of all suffering. The Sage Patanjali refers to these ailments as the five kleshas. These are classified as beings of ignorance, ego, attachment, attachment to others, hatred, and fear of death (Avidya, Asmita, Raga, Dvesha, Abhinivesa). The first step toward achieving eternal bliss is realizing and acknowledging the existence of these klesha inside oneself. These klesha offer a glimpse into the mind. Warfare throughout history and the current state of human misery are the outcomes of raga and dvesha. Before acting, one should think clearly and view the situation through the lens of klesha. This leads in deeds, rather than regret and sorrow. Chitta Prasadanam, a lovely formula provided by Sage Patanjali, can be used to make decisions that lead to bliss. "Blissful Mind" is the literal translation of Chitta Prasadanam. The great sage also provided a straightforward, tiered strategy to help everyone experience this joy.

All we need to do is practice camaraderie (maitri), compassion (karuna), and joy (mudita), and cultivate apathy toward pleasure (sukha), pain (dukha), virtue (punya), and nastiness (apunya). One can acquire chitta prasadanam, the blissful and tranquil condition of chitta (mind), by repeatedly adopting this attitude.

Only the practice of pranayama (breath control), guided by a qualified teacher, can accomplish this. You can attain mental clarity through pranayama. All that is left to do is change your bad emotions into positive ones. For instance, when one of your friends succeeds, do not be envious of them or try to find fault; instead, really celebrate their achievement. In addition to making you happy, this also wins you a lifelong buddy. The contrary is also true; when someone is grieving, be compassionate and helpful. Increase someone's happiness when they are experiencing a happy time by telling others about their accomplishments; this will make them feel even happier.

1.1 What is chitta?

According to Samkhya philosophy (25 elements theory), the Chitta is the combination of Manas (mind), Buddhi (intellect), and Ahamkara (ego) [1]. Trigunas are also a part of the Chitta, which is the origin of human consciousness. The proportion of Sattva, Rajas, and Tamas in the Chitta varies from time to time and determines how an individual acts and perceives the world, as well as their intelligence. Trigunas are responsible for our fluctuating emotions, which range from being restless and lethargic to being very active and curious about things.

2. Need of purification/cleansing of chitta?

The sutra on Chitta Prasadana is after the sutra on Chitta Vikshepa (disturbances of mind). Patanjali explains that disturbances of mind could be in form of sadness, disappointment, anger, imbalance in breathing, etc. and is caused by nine kinds of Antarayas (distractions) that occur on a yogi's journey to self-attainment [2].

2.1 Panch klesha

The only way we can achieve enlightenment or samadhi is by defeating these five challenges. We are unable to advance past the physical body when we interact with the pancha klesha, which keeps us bound to earthly afflictions. Recognizing and comprehending these mental afflictions can aid us in returning to our genuine nature because our truest selves are free from this klesha.

Of these five challenges, avidya is likely the most significant because ignorance makes it difficult to identify the other ills. The most severe form of suffering results from our ignorance of our true nature because it fosters a sense of alienation from all other beings. A strong sense of our interconnectedness with the universe, as well as our inherent traits of calm and compassion, are necessary for overcoming avidya.

Ignorance gives rise to a dualistic view of oneself and the world. Asmita, or egoism, is a dominant sense of I, Me, and I. We lose sight of the fact that everything is interconnected, that our actions affect others as well as ourselves. Strong attachments to people, locations, and roles are also brought on by egoism. When we are emotionally invested in our wishes, we experience intense hunger, or rage, which causes suffering when things do not turn out exactly how we want them to.

Aversion, or the persistent desire to turn away from the things we find unpleasant, is the result of being controlled by need. This fosters a lingering, nagging sensation of unhappiness and is dvesha. It is only normal for us to dread change when we have this kind of mix of attachments, desires, and aversions. This struggle for survival—abhinivesha—is the last barrier. We can only completely free ourselves from pain when we can let go of control and accept impermanence.

DOI: http://dx.doi.org/10.5772/intechopen.1002797

2.2 Yoga antaraya

Yoga's nine key challenges are:

Vyadhi - Physical or mental illness or disease. If you are physically ill, practicing yoga is challenging. To prevent sickness and promote good health, it is crucial to have a healthy lifestyle.

Styana: Lack of interest in carrying out one's kartavya or duty. By putting off our practice and making up reasons to not be on the path and complete the work, we procrastinate.

Sanshaya is the act of doubting one's abilities or the effects of yoga. According to the Brihad-ranyaka-Upanishad (4.4.23), we can only know Reality once we are free of uncertainty. It is crucial to develop faith in both the yoga path and one.

Pramada: A lack of persistence, carelessness, and heedlessness. Yoga is a science and an art and doing it improperly can have unpredictable effects that could even be harmful.

Alasya: Inertia of the body or mind brought on by the dominance of the tamasic element. Yoga's path involves self-control, ardor, and tapas (willpower). You will not reach your full potential if you are lazy.

Affection for enjoyable goods and overindulgence. If we want to advance in yoga, we must learn to "let go" of our ties to desires and material things.

False vision and hasty assurance are both examples of bhrantidarshan. The formation of an incorrect belief about yoga practice and its results can cause injury and disappointment in addition to taking one off the path of yoga.

Non-attainment of the following yogic level or accomplishment is known as aladdha-bhumikatva. This occurs because of incorrect or subpar practice, which gives the impression that one is "stuck" and inspires discouragement.

Anawasthitatwa: An unstable or transient stage or achievement in yoga. Being unable to retain an accomplished level can be quite frustrating. Again, improper or subpar practice may be to blame [3].

3. Chitta prasadanam

Chitta Prasadanam, as prescribed by Maharishi Patanjali in his famous Yoga Sutras, is valuable wisdom that can help us maintain a peaceful and beautiful state of mind, regardless of the actions of others. Chitta in yoga is defined as the mind-stuff and *Prasadanam* means the act of making something pure and beautiful.

मैत्रीकरुणामुदितोपेक्षाणां सुखदुःखपुण्यापुण्यविषयाणां भावनातः चित्तप्रसादनम् ॥३३॥.

Maitrikarunamuditopeksanam.

sukhaduhkhapunyapunyavisayanam.

bhavanataschittaprasadanam (1/33 PYS) [4].

Maitri: friendliness; karuna: compassion; Mudita; gladness; upeksanam: indifference; sukha: happiness; duhkha: misery; punya: virtue; apunya: vice; visayanam: of the objects; bhavanatah: attitude; chitta: mind; prasadanam: purification, making peace.

By practicing the attitudes of friendliness, compassion, gladness, and indifference in response to happiness, misery, virtue, and vice, the mind becomes pure and at peace.

Without first purifying, or making the mind tranquil in nature, it is impossible to develop focus. This sutra illustrates the ideal method for doing this. It is a technique for developing a kind, compassionate, joyful, and unconcerned attitude toward those or things that bring happiness, suffering, virtue, or vice. By upholding this mentality—friendliness toward the joyful, compassion toward the miserable, joy regarding the righteous, and indifference toward those who are full of vice—the aspirant's mind is liberated from disruptive forces, and as a result, it is at peace.

According to the sutra, practicing the four mental virtues namely, Maitri, Karuna, Mudita, and Upeshka is the ultimate way to experience the calmness of the mind.

3.1 Maitri—friendliness

Maitri could be understood as the feeling of friendliness or loving-kindness. So, this part of the sutra suggests developing kind and friendly thoughts toward the happiness of people.

We all know people who could be more blessed than us—be it in terms of wealth, beauty, or possessions. And oftentimes we end up comparing ourselves to them.

Maharishi Patanjali teaches us to regain our peace of mind by developing friendly thoughts toward happier people, instead of allowing insecure thoughts to enter our mind.

The renowned yogi Swami Vivekananda interprets it as having friendly thoughts toward all fellow human beings; after all, we are part of one cosmos and connected to each other in a way.

3.2 Karuna—compassion

Karuna is the attitude of compassion toward other people's sorrows. This part of the sutra teaches us to develop loving compassion toward people who are in pain or suffering.

The mind may be accustomed to being indifferent toward other people's pain because it is not our own. Or we could feel pity for people who are not as blessed as us. But the feeling of pity only separates us from them.

Instead, training the mind to feel genuine compassion and concern toward others enables us to connect with them and our higher self eventually.

3.3 Mudita—joy

Mudita means joy or delight. This part of the sutra teaches us to develop gladness over the good deeds and achievements of others, instead of allowing envious feelings to take over our mind.

Jealousy is a vice that can easily plague us when we hear of others' achievements. In fact, the human mind can look for flaws even in the most virtuous people.

While it may not be natural for us to feel elated over a neighbor or colleague's achievements, we do feel joyous over the achievements of our close ones. The difference is that we experience the happiness of only those who we feel connected with.

We must remind ourselves that we are all connected in this world. And feeling genuinely happy for all others, devoid of any envy, allows the divine peace to flow within us.

3.4 Upeksha—apunya

The word *Upeksha* is displaying indifference or neutrality toward negative behavior or vices of others. And this may be the toughest part of practicing.

Let us admit, it takes deliberate effort to not act judgmental toward others. The mind can cling on to the mistakes made by others and look for opportunities to correct them.

Maharishi Patanjali advocates exactly the opposite of this habit — to show acceptance or "equanimity" toward wrong actions [5]. An easy way to instill this habit is by reminding ourselves that we all make mistakes while being unaware of them. Others could be doing the same. We must let our mind accept that "simply overlooking other people's wrongdoings" is the prescribed way to finding peace according to our ancient scriptures.

4. Mental wellbeing

According to the World Health Organization (WHO), mental health is "a state of well-being in which the individual realizes his or her own abilities, can cope with the normal stresses of life, can work productively and fruitfully, and is able to make a contribution to his or her community [6]."

When it identifies positive feelings and positive functioning as essential components of mental health, this definition raises several questions and lends itself to potential misunderstandings, even though it represents a significant advancement in moving away from the conceptualization of mental health as a state of absence of mental illness.

It is challenging to reconcile the multiple challenging living situations in which well-being may even be ill with the idea that well-being is a fundamental component of mental health. For instance, most people would consider it mentally unhealthy for someone to feel at ease while killing several people during a war operation, but they would consider it good for someone to feel desperate after losing their job in an atmosphere with limited work alternatives [7].

People with good mental health experience depression, illness, rage, or other negative emotions regularly; this is a necessary component of leading a full life. Despite this, mental health is commonly perceived as a completely good condition marked by joyful emotions and environmental control.

5. Yoga antraya and chitta prasadanam remedies to enhance mental health

When the devotees of yoga practice yoga, then according to the rituals, some obstacles arise, which can be of physical and mental level. These obstacles block the path of yoga, due to which the practice of yoga gets obstructed. Maharishi Patanjali describes Antaraya in the context of the obstacles that end because of contemplation of God's name and form and explains how the seeker can end these obstacles and purify his mind. Maharshi Patanjali describes nine types of obstacles and describes the other five sub-obstacles that happen along with them. To remove those obstacles, he describes various measures according to the ability of the seeker. These obstacles are called Yogantraya and the way to remove them is called the way of Chitta Prasadanam. Antaraya means disturbances or distractions, that is, whatever distractions occur in the mind, it causes distractions and creates the barrier in the path of Yoga that leads to the Samadhi.

> *Vyadhi-Styana-Samsaya-Pramada-Alasya-Avirati-Bhrantidarsana-Alabdhabhumikatva-Anavasthitatvani-Cittaviksepah-Te-Antarayah (Patanjali Yoga Sutra 1/30) [8]*

Vyadhi: disease, illness, sickness
Styana: inefficiency, dullness
Samsaya: indecision, doubt
Pramada: carelessness, negligence
Alasaya: sloth, laziness
Avirati: sensuality, craving
Bhranti darsana: false views or perception
Alabdhabhumikatva: failing to attain stages of practice
Anavasthitatvani: inability to maintain
Cittaviksepah: distractions of the mind
Te: they are
Antarayah: obstacles, impediments

According to Swami Hariharanand Aranya- With Ishwar Pranidhan, all these obstacles are removed.

According to Vigyanbhikshu, those who disturb the mind are called Antaraya. Interruptions are visible in the presence of mind-sets due to their disturbance. Due to being nutritious to the body, the dissimilar imbalance of Vata, Kapha, and Pitta, the juices resulting from diet and the eyes and mind, etc., is called disease. Once' inability to perform yoga rituals is called inactivity. Mental inactivity is called styana. Ambivalent knowledge is called doubt. It is foolish not to research the means of samadhi. Due to Kaphadi, there is physical gravity and due to Tamoguna, there is mental gravity. Laziness is the root cause of sadhaka's inability to practice the ritual of samadhi due to these two reasons. The attachment derived from the closeness of the subject is called avarati. Having opposite knowledge about the substance certified by the Acharyas is delusion. Not getting even a single piece of land like Madhumati etc., even after performing the rituals of the means of attaining yoga, is the absence of land. The loss of concentration due to the instability of the mind after attaining any of the Madhumatyadi lands is called non-existence.

According to Swami Vivekananda, this body is the only boat to go across this sea of life. One whose body is unwell cannot be a Yogi. When mental inertia sets in, all our interest in yoga is lost. And in the absence of this interest, there will be neither determination nor strength to do spiritual practice. No matter how strong our thought-generated belief in this subject may be, until there are supernatural experiences like Doordarshan, etc., many doubts will be present about the veracity of this knowledge. When all these are realized little by little, then the seeker becomes even more diligent in the path of meditation. While doing sadhana, you will see that for a few days or a few weeks, the mind becomes concentrated and stable without any effort, but suddenly this source of progress has stopped, do not lose your perseverance.

According to Swami Omanandatirtha - These nine obstacles are removed from concentration.

According to Pandit. Shriram Sharma Acharya - Obstacle to a seeker walking on the path of Yoga. Those who lead astray are of nine types-

1. (Vyadhi) Disease- Any kind of disease in the body, weakness in the senses and anxiety etc. in the mingles a disease.

2. (Styan) - Being unable to work, inaction, discouragement in work or lack of ability is called styan.

3. (Sanshaya) Doubt- Not having faith in the objective condition of Yogavidya and doubting the success of one's efforts is called doubt.

4. (Pramada)Negligence-Doing yoga carelessly, leaving the routine incomplete and not worrying about it even if it gets spoiled is called Pramad.

5. (Alasya) Laziness- due to the presence of Tamoguna, the body remains healthy, but excess of tamoguna leads to the tendency that will not let us engage in work.

6. (Avirati) - due to being attached to the subject, the mind remains attached to the objects and the lack of disinterest in the mind is called avirati.

7. (Bhranti Darshana) Illusion- Due to some reason of lack of knowledge, there is no knowledge of the philosophy and means of spirituality or this means is not suitable, such illusory knowledge is called illusion.

8. (Alabdha-bhumikatva)- Not being able to reach the state of a seeker even after doing continuous meditation and the speed of mind getting blocked in the middle is called alabdha bhumikatva.

9. (Anavastitha) - The inability of mind to remain concentrated or steady, due to which it cannot reach the role and because of instability, the wavering of the mind is called anavasthiti.

These are the nine kinds of obstacles that interrupt peace of mind and lead toward the mental health degradation.

6. Conclusion

Chitta Prasadanam is an ancient technique that was used by the Yogis for the purification and stability of the mind so that they can pursue the Yogic practice with the excellence or without any distraction. Nowadays this practice is very beneficial not only to attain the state of samadhi but to achieve good mental health. The lives of almost every individual have become hectic due to numerous reasons. In this cutting-edge period, an enormous extent of populace adjusting current culture like stationary lifestyle, amount, and nature of food, abandoning their practice, way of life. Today, most of the individuals are prepared to think twice about their prosperity to accomplish more significant standards to adapt up with the cultural strain their way of life put on them, subsequently stress has turned into our steady friend. Apart from stress, there are numerous factors which are affecting our mental health. If we practice the Chitta Prasadanam, then we can modify our thoughts, be able to give positive direction to our thoughts so that we can be in the state of mental peace. It is a very simple rule that if our mind is at peace every other thing can be at peace. Ultimately each one of us is doing work just for satisfaction or for the mental peace. If we can pursue the four feelings "Maitri, Karuna, Mudita, and Upeksha," then we can transform other negative feelings "guilt, greed, envy, jealousy, etc.," and can save our mind from the several mental illnesses.

Author details

Deepshikha Thakur
ITM University, Gwalior, India

*Address all correspondence to: tdeepshikha7@gmail.com

References

[1] Rao KR. The gunas of prakrti according to the samkhya philosophy. Philosophy East and West. 1963;**13**(1):61

[2] Saraswati SS. Four Chapters on Freedom. Commentary on Patanjali Yoga Sutra. Munger, Bihar, India: Yoga Publication Trust; 2013. pp. 29-31

[3] Iyenger BKS. Light on Yoga Sutras of Patanjali. UP, India: Harper Collins Publishers; 2011

[4] Ranganathan S. Patanjali's yoga sutra. UK: Penguin; 2008

[5] Iyengar BK. Light on the Yoga Sutras of Patanjali. Aquarian/Thorsons; 1993

[6] van Agteren J, Iasiello M, Lo L, Bartholomaeus J, Kopsaftis Z, Carey M, et al. A systematic review and meta-analysis of psychological interventions to improve mental wellbeing. Nature Human Behaviour. 2021;**5**(5):631-652

[7] Baik C, Larcombe W, Brooker A. How universities can enhance student mental wellbeing: The student perspective. Higher Education Research & Development. 2019;**38**(4):674-687

[8] Miller BS. Yoga: Discipline of Freedom: The Yoga Sutra Attributed to Patanjali. University of California Press; 1996

Chapter 2

Exploring the Multidimensional Health Effects of Yogasana: A Comprehensive Overview

Sobika Rao and Rameswar Pal

Abstract

The term "Yoga" is derived from the Sanskrit root "Yuj," which translates to "to join," "to yoke," or "to unite." Its global appeal stems from its evidence-based holistic approach. Today, a robust scientific consensus exists on the therapeutic benefits of Yoga, supported by a burgeoning body of research. Various Yogic practices, including asana (physical postures), pranayama (breath control), and dhyana (meditation), offer multifaceted health advantages. Yogasana, a cornerstone of Yoga, integrates physical postures with controlled breathing techniques to enhance physiological, psychological, and emotional well-being. As the third limb of Ashtanga Yoga, Yogasana yields diverse physiological effects, from cellular modulation to systemic improvements across the human body. Sukshma vyama, a subset of Yogasana, promotes localized blood circulation and facilitates articulation in synovial joints, thereby optimizing biomechanical alignment and mitigating muscular imbalances. Moreover, Yogasana induces slower, deeper breathing patterns, eliciting a predominant activation of the parasympathetic nervous system, which is crucial for stress management in modern society. Specific asanas stimulate digestive functions, facilitating the absorption and elimination of metabolic waste products, thereby fostering gastrointestinal health and optimizing the gut-brain axis. This chapter offers a comprehensive synthesis of scientific literature elucidating the physiological and psychological effects of Yogasana practice, providing an empirically grounded understanding of its therapeutic potential.

Keywords: yoga, asana, health, performance, biomechanics

1. Introduction

Yogasanas find first place in "*Hath Yoga pradipika*" and third place in "*Patanjali Ashtang Yoga*." Asanas constitute a vital aspect of Yoga, although there is a common misconception that Yoga solely revolves around physical postures. However, it is imperative to distinguish asanas from mere postures or exercises, as the former entails a conscious integration of breath awareness. While assuming a specific posture, one's mind may wander, but the practice of asanas necessitates focused attention.

Presently, a substantial portion of scientific inquiry is directed toward unraveling the effects of Yogasanas. In this discourse, an attempt has been made to examine the physiological and psychological impacts of various Yogasanas comprehensively.

In Patanjali's Yoga-darsan an asana is defined as – sthiram sukham asanam. 'स्थिरसुखमसनम् I. 'According to Patanjali, "steady and comfortable posture is asana" [1]. Any posture that can be maintained with comfort is an asana.

2. Classification of asanas

As per traditional texts, the asanas can be classified mainly into 03 categories [2–4]:

1. Cultural Asanas

2. Relaxative Asanas

3. Meditative Asanas

2.1 Cultural asana

This category represents diverse asanas that offer a comprehensive approach to the physiological and psychological well-being of an individual. These asanas serve as foundational practices, priming individuals for more advanced Yogic techniques. They entail dynamic movements involving various joints around multiple anatomical axes and planes, including flexion–extension, abduction–adduction, and external–internal rotation. Performed in various positions such as standing, kneeling, sitting, prone lying, and supine lying, each asana imposes unique physical and biomechanical demands, contributing to the complexity of the practice. From a physiological standpoint, these asanas are instrumental in fortifying the musculoskeletal system through static stretching, which enhances muscle tone and flexibility. Notably, they optimize spinal column mobility, facilitating maximal vertebral movement. Moreover, these practices elicit profound effects on visceral organs within the thoracic and abdominal cavities by modulating intra-abdominal pressure. This regulation supports the proper functioning of vital organs, thereby promoting overall health and vitality [2–4].

2.2 Relaxative asanas

Asanas that place the body in a lying position—either supine or prone—are considered relaxing asanas. When lying down, the body is entirely supported on a surface, making it the most accessible position to maintain with the least amount of muscle work needed. For example, in Savasana, all postural muscles can relax because the back surface of the body becomes the base of support (BOS). The lowest center of gravity (COG) is found in Savasana.

Therefore, poses intended to promote relaxation are made such that no muscles are tensed, or there is no need to maintain specific body positions. Since these asanas facilitate easy prana (vital energy) flow, they are necessary for total relaxation. The two popular poses for relaxation are Makarasana and Shavasana [2–4].

2.3 Meditative asanas

As a practice, meditation includes focused introspection while in one's physical space. Attaining both mental and physical stability is essential to reach such focus. Therefore, meditative asanas are those poses that guarantee optimal spinal column alignment while providing a broad and stable base of support (BOS). These qualities are essential prerequisites to practicing advanced yogic techniques like Dhyana and Pranayama.

When performing meditative asanas, practitioners attempt to hold the pose for prolonged periods of time, sometimes up to several hours. This long duration makes it easier to conduct longer sessions of higher forms of Yoga, such as Dhyana and Pranayama, which involve withdrawing from outside stimuli and cultivating perfect stillness and comfort, e.g., Padmasana, Sidhhasana [2–4].

2.4 Phases of asanas

According to Sherrington, posture is intrinsically linked to movement, akin to a shadow following its object. This assertion underscores the notion that motion commences and concludes within a given position. The point of origin for any movement is termed the starting position. Five fundamental starting positions exist, from which all others derive: standing, kneeling, sitting, lying, and hanging. Stability and equilibrium within these positions are upheld by the equilibrium of forces exerted upon the body. Muscular contraction is executed isometrically when it is employed to maintain this equilibrium and stability, signifying that the muscle length remains unchanged during contraction [2–4].

Each asana commences from a distinct starting point. Every conceivable asana initiates from a specific initial posture and concludes by reverting back to this initial posture. The different phases of asanas are as follows:

1. Starting Position

2. Moving into an asana (dynamic muscle contraction)

3. Holding that asana as per the individual's capacity (isometric muscle contraction)

4. Moving out of the asana (dynamic muscle contraction)

5. Getting back into the starting position.

Some examples of asansa which have standing as a starting position are TĀḌĀSANA, VṚKṢĀSANA, ARDHA CAKRĀSANA, etc.

Some examples of asansa which have sitting as a starting position are VAJRĀSANA, ARDHA UṢṬRĀSANA, UTTĀNA MANDŪKĀSANA, etc.

Some examples of asansa which have prone lying as a starting position are MAKARĀSANA, BHUJAṄGĀSANA, ŚALABHĀSANA, etc.

Some examples of asansa which have supine lying as a starting position, are SETUBANDHĀSANA, ARDHA HALĀSANA, PAVANA MUKTĀSANA, etc.

3. General guidelines for the practice of yoga asana

The Ashtanga Yoga of Maharshi Patanjali outlines eight branches of yoga; practicing asanas is the third and necessary step in the yoga path. For this reason, it is crucial to understand the concepts of Yama and Niyama before performing any asana [2–4].

1. Asanas should be performed with individuals advised to seek guidance from a medical professional or therapist, particularly if they have underlying medical conditions.

2. It is essential for the bladder and bowels to be empty before commencing the practice of asanas.

3. The execution of asanas should be characterized by a relaxed demeanor, ensuring stability, comfort, and a sense of effortlessness.

4. The duration of holding the final pose should align with the practitioner's capabilities, emphasizing individual capacity.

5. Abrupt and forceful movements during transitions into and out of asanas should be avoided to mitigate the risk of injury.

6. Optimal practice entails maintaining each posture for a minimum of 10 seconds or at least three complete breath cycles.

7. Prior knowledge of the indications and contraindications associated with each asana is essential for practitioners to ensure safe and effective practice.

8. A bath is recommended after 20–30 min following the conclusion of a yoga session.

9. Consumption of food is advised only after 20–30 min post-yoga practice, allowing the body ample time to transition and restore equilibrium.

4. Impacts of yogasana on the human body

The human body consists of trillions of cells, which combine to form tissues, and tissues combine to form organs. These organs, in turn, assemble into organ systems, ultimately constituting the entirety of an individual organism. Within the human body, numerous systems operate in harmony to sustain life and overall function. A fundamental grasp of human anatomy and physiology is crucial for comprehending the body's internal mechanisms and how various yogic practices influence different layers of existence, known as koshas.

Although the term "Yogaasanas" implies movement, it is often mistakenly believed to impact the musculoskeletal system primarily. However, yogic postures exert substantial effects on various vital organs and systems beyond just the musculoskeletal system. These systems encompass the nervous system, musculoskeletal system, respiratory system, cardiovascular system, digestive system, excretory system, reproductive system, lymphatic system, endocrine system, and integumentary system.

5. Biomechanical impact of yogasanas

The musculoskeletal system plays a vital role in maintaining body structure, facilitating movement, and safeguarding essential organs. Engaging in regular practice of Yogasanas is widely acknowledged for its positive impact on musculoskeletal health. Understanding the mechanics behind performing yoga asanas is crucial. Essentially, yoga asanas entail movement, which primarily occurs at the joints due to skeletal muscle contractions along specific planes and axes within the body. Human anatomy recognizes three principal anatomical planes: frontal, sagittal, and transverse, which correspond to forward/backward, side-to-side, and rotatory movements, respectively. Moreover, the range of motion (ROM) in various synovial joints is influenced by multiple factors, including anatomical structure and individual flexibility. Alignment in yoga asanas refers to how body segments are positioned in relation to each other, as each asana imposes its unique physical demands. Optimal alignment entails movement across all three planes and around all three axes of the body. Additionally, the stability of a particular asana hinges on three critical factors: the center of gravity (COG), the line of gravity (LOG), and the base of support (BOS). These elements vary across different asanas, resulting in varying degrees of stability and physical demand.

Properly executed asanas play a pivotal role in preserving musculoskeletal integrity. When performed with correct alignment, Yogasanas contribute to enhancing muscle flexibility and optimizing joint range of motion. These practices facilitate movement across all three anatomical planes and axes, thereby mitigating muscle imbalances resulting from factors such as poor posture, prolonged sedentary behavior, or ergonomic deficiencies in work environments. Regular engagement in Yogasanas also fosters bone health by adhering to Wolff's Law, which posits that bone formation is directly influenced by mechanical stress and strain. Through weight-bearing Yogasanas, bone strengthening and mineralization are stimulated, thereby enhancing bone density and resilience. These weight-loading practices can mitigate age-related bone loss, bolster bone density, and avert conditions like osteoporosis [5].

When executed with precise alignment, standing asanas preserve the spine's physiological curvature and enhance posture. Each asana imposes distinct biomechanical demands, resulting in selective stretching of specific muscle groups while concurrently activating others to accommodate increased demand. This dynamic movement creates a symbiotic relationship wherein specific muscles undergo elongation, promoting flexibility, while opposing muscle groups experience intensified activity, fostering tonicity and strength. Consequently, a harmonious equilibrium is sustained between the flexibility and strength of agonist and antagonist muscle pairs during the execution of individual asanas. Yogasanas exhibit promising potential in augmenting core muscle strength in practitioners [6, 7].

Hence, it can be concluded that musculoskeletal ailments and occupational afflictions are increasingly prevalent in modern society, posing significant health burdens. Integrating Yoga into comprehensive treatment strategies can offer substantial benefits for managing and mitigating musculoskeletal disorders. Yoga, a holistic mind-body practice, amalgamates physical postures, controlled breathing, meditation, and relaxation techniques. This multifaceted approach fosters enhancements in flexibility, strength, balance, and somatic awareness, concurrently promoting mental well-being. Moreover, Yoga augments local circulation, facilitating the elimination of metabolic byproducts and oxidative stress, thereby ameliorating discomfort and expediting tissue repair processes. Emphasizing proper joint alignment, Yogasanas cultivate strength within postural musculature by sustaining optimal alignment over extended durations. This methodical approach to alignment and muscular engagement forms a foundational aspect of Yoga practice, contributing to its therapeutic efficacy in addressing musculoskeletal issues [8].

6. Impacts of yogaasana on the respiratory system

Consistent engagement in yogic routines heightens respiratory efficiency, diminishing the susceptibility to respiratory infections, augmenting lung capacity, and refining breathing patterns. The sustained practice of Yoga diminishes the likelihood of respiratory ailments such as asthma and chronic obstructive pulmonary disease (COPD) [6]. Yogic practices enhance various lung volumes and capacities, including tidal volume, vital capacity, maximum ventilator volume, and forced vital capacity. Different types of breathing maneuvers during the practice of asanas exert influence on respiration by voluntary modification of breathing patterns through regulation of higher brain centers. Respiration, involving muscular contraction and thoracic cage movement, is impacted by specific asanas with stretching effects on the chest wall. These postures, such as Tadasana, Trikonasana, Bhujangasana, and Dhanurasana, contribute to the expansion of the chest wall, maintenance of spinal curvature, and correction of postural defects. Consequently, this aligned posture fosters deeper respiration. Yogic practices further augment the vital capacity of practitioners while reducing respiratory rate. This enhancement is facilitated by the expansion of the chest area, leading to increased anteroposterior and vertical dimensions of the thoracic cavity, thereby accommodating more air within the lungs. Isometric contraction of respiratory muscles during yogic techniques enhances muscle strength, particularly in chest muscles like the diaphragm and intercostals. This strengthening effect positively impacts lung function parameters such as forced vital capacity, forced expiratory volume at the end of the first second, maximum voluntary ventilation, peak expiratory flow rate, and breath-holding time prolongation [9, 10]. The practice of asanas enhances circulation, thereby facilitating adequate blood flow to essential organs. Consistent engagement in yogic asanas and pranayamas, as a non-pharmacological intervention for individuals with ailments, holds promise for enhancing pulmonary function overall [11].

7. Impacts of yogasana on the cardiovascular system

Yogic asanas, characterized by dynamic and static postures, exert diverse effects on the cardiovascular system. Emerging research indicates that specific asanas possess the ability to induce relaxation by eliciting reductions in heart rate, blood pressure, and sympathetic nervous system activity. Conversely, vigorous asanas can elevate heart rate and activate the cardiovascular system. Across the spectrum of asana practice, sukshmvayama, the warmup practices consistently promote increased blood flow to the targeted areas. Clinical investigations demonstrate that regular yogic practices contribute to improvements in blood pressure, lipid profile, and overall cardiovascular resilience. Notably, Savasana, characterized by minimal muscle engagement and mental relaxation, facilitates a state of general relaxation. This relaxation response is accompanied by a reduction in muscle tone and a shift toward parasympathetic dominance, resulting in significant reductions in basal heart rate and systemic blood pressure. Engaging in yogasanas fosters enhanced circulation, augments venous return, and elevates cardiac output (including stroke and minute volume). Furthermore, yogic practices contribute to toning cardiac muscles and reducing systolic and diastolic blood pressure, promoting cardiovascular health and function [12, 13]. However, certain asanas have specific contraindications, particularly inverted poses like Sarvangasana, Viparita Karni, Halasana, and Mayurasana. These poses should be avoided or performed under medical supervision by individuals with hypertension.

8. Impact of yogaasanas on the cardiorespiratory performance

The positive effects of yoga asanas on the cardiorespiratory system are rooted in diverse physiological and neurological processes. These include the regulation of the autonomic nervous system, alterations in baroreflex sensitivity, and enhancements in respiratory muscle coordination. A more profound comprehension of these mechanisms offers valuable insights for incorporating yoga asanas into holistic cardiorespiratory rehabilitation and preventive strategies [14].

The consistent engagement in specific yogasanas has been linked to notable enhancements in cardiopulmonary fitness. Asanas demanding prolonged exertion and regulated respiration are observed to augment aerobic capacity and general endurance levels. Moreover, yogic disciplines contribute to improved physical performance across various metrics, encompassing aerobic capacity, anaerobic power, body composition, and cardiovascular endurance [15, 16].

9. Impacts of yogasana on the digestive system

Poses involving abdominal twists can stimulate and massage vital organs such as the liver, pancreas, gallbladder, and various parts of the digestive tract. This manipulation potentially promotes better digestion, enhances nutrient absorption, and may contribute to overall gastrointestinal health [17].

It is widely acknowledged that serotonin, a neurotransmitter crucial for mood regulation, is influenced in part by the digestive tract. Dysfunction of the "gut-brain" axis or enteric nervous system is linked with gastrointestinal disturbances such as irritable bowel syndrome (IBS), alongside mental health disorders like depression and anxiety. Yoga promotes a harmonious interaction between the mind and body, significantly improving digestion and mood regulation [18–20].

The described concept elucidates how emotional states can influence the functioning of digestive organs, resulting in issues such as acidity, indigestion, and gastric disturbances. Practically all yoga asanas impact the body's digestive system by enhancing processes such as digestion, absorption, and secretion, as well as relieving constipation, optimizing peristaltic movement, regulating juice secretion, and improving blood circulation to abdominal organs. Furthermore, the abdominal wall provides support to the abdominal viscera, thereby aiding in maintaining the tone of smooth muscles within the viscera. Specific asanas exemplify these effects. Vajrasana, particularly effective post-meal, aids in proper digestion, facilitates the release of Apana Vayu and alleviates indigestion and constipation. Padmasana enhances blood flow in the abdominal region, benefiting internal organs and digestion. Trikonasana massages and tones all internal digestive organs, enhancing appetite and the efficiency of the digestive system. Stress plays a significant role in disrupting digestive function. Yoga practices, encompassing both asanas and relaxation techniques, have been scientifically proven to mitigate stress levels and foster a sense of calmness. This relationship between stress reduction through yoga and its positive impacts on digestion underscores the holistic benefits of yoga for both mental and physical well-being [21].

Certain yogasanas entail controlled movements involving gentle twists, compressions, and stretches, strategically targeting the abdominal organs, including the stomach, liver, and pancreas. These specific movements have been observed to elicit physiological responses that enhance digestive enzyme secretion, facilitate gastric emptying, and improve overall digestive efficiency. Asanas emphasizing forward bends and controlled abdominal contractions have demonstrated the ability to modulate gut motility positively. Regular incorporation of such practices into one's routine may offer preventive benefits against constipation and promote the maintenance of optimal bowel function. Yoga has garnered recognition as an adjunctive therapy for a spectrum of gastrointestinal disorders, encompassing irritable bowel syndrome (IBS), acid reflux, and inflammatory bowel disease (IBD). Through the utilization of targeted yoga asanas and breathing methodologies, symptomatology associated with these conditions can be mitigated, while concurrently addressing stressors that often exacerbate symptoms. This holistic approach to management holds promises for enhancing the overall quality of life for individuals grappling with gastrointestinal disorders [19, 22].

The enteric nervous system, also known as the intrinsic nervous system, constitutes a fundamental division of the peripheral nervous system responsible for regulating the digestive tract's function. These mechanisms may include the stimulation of the vagus nerve, modulation of the gut-brain axis, and the relaxation response. Understanding these mechanisms can provide insights into integrating yoga asanas as a complementary approach to digestive health management.

10. Impacts of yogasana on nervous system

Regular engagement in yogic practices exhibits notable benefits for cognitive function, sleep quality, and brain structure. Specifically, the practice of Hatha Yoga appears to be correlated with facilitating neuroplastic changes within executive brain systems, as evidenced by an augmentation in gray matter volume. This consistent yogic regimen is also associated with heightened gamma-aminobutyric acid (GABA) secretion, regulation of dopamine levels, and increased serotonin secretion. A single session of yoga asanas has been demonstrated to elevate the levels of gamma-aminobutyric acid in practitioners. GABA, functioning as a neurotransmitter, induces a state of relaxation by mitigating symptoms associated with stress and anxiety. Prior research has underscored the capacity of yoga asanas to enhance GABA levels, consequently eliciting a relaxed physiological state [22, 23]. Yoga exerts beneficial effects on neurotransmitter levels in practitioners, including the enhancement of dopamine and serotonin. Elevated dopamine levels contribute to reduced risk of Parkinson's disease and improved coordination. Meanwhile, serotonin serves as a biochemical indicator of happiness, enhancing mood and counteracting depression when levels are sufficient. Yogic practices additionally reduce cortisol levels, a biomarker of stress, and enhance alpha (α) wave activity in electroencephalography, indicating heightened states of relaxation. Furthermore, yoga enhances sleep quality. Notably, yoga practice has been associated with increased levels of Brain-Derived Neurotrophic Factor (BDNF), crucial for adult neurogenesis, as well as oxytocin.

These neurochemicals play pivotal roles in cognition, further underscoring the cognitive benefits conferred by yogasana practice [19, 24, 25]. BDNF and serotonin exert regulatory influence over crucial processes in the adult brain, including neurogenesis, synaptic plasticity, and neuronal viability. The practice of yoga exerts multifaceted effects on the autonomic nervous system (ANS), higher cognitive functions, and mental well-being. Clinical studies have provided evidence supporting the capacity of yoga asanas to modulate the ANS, promoting parasympathetic dominance, reducing blood pressure and heart rate, facilitating relaxation, and fostering approach-oriented behaviors [26, 27].

11. Impacts of yogasana on endocrine system

The endocrine system consists of glands that pour their secretion directly into the bloodstream. The hormone is a chemical substance that influences the target cells' function. They are of two types: water-soluble and fat-soluble. The endocrine system is vital for maintaining homeostasis of the human body, i.e., maintaining a constant internal environment in response to internal and external stressors. The nervous system is also essential to maintain homeostasis and is rapidly acting. However, the endocrine system is slower and has a long-lasting control than the nervous system.

The internal environment is tightly controlled; this reasonably constant state is called homeostasis. When this balance is disturbed in response to various stressors (internal and external), there is a severe risk to the individual's well-being. Some essential physiological variables maintained within narrow limits by homeostatic control mechanisms are core temperature, body fluids' pH (acidity or alkalinity), blood glucose levels, etc. Homeostasis is maintained using feedback mechanisms (negative and positive feedback mechanisms). The various endocrine glands are pituitary gland, thyroid gland, parathyroid gland, adrenal gland, pancreas, and gonads.

Yoga fine tunes the different inter-related links of the hypothalamic-pituitary-adrenal (HPA) axis, which helps to keep the mind and body of the practitioner aligned and relaxed and leads to optimal functioning of the endocrine system by reducing the effects of various stressors, which brings about a change in the internal environment of the body. Yogic practices decrease stress by modulating the HPA axis [19]. It regulates the thyroid hormone secretion to maintain balance and metabolism [28].

12. Impact of yogasana on renal physiology

The kidneys play a crucial role in preserving fluid and electrolyte balance, eliminating waste products, and regulating blood pressure. Yogasanas are integral for supporting renal health, as certain poses can enhance blood circulation to the kidneys, potentially improving renal filtration and waste elimination. Consistent practice of specific yoga asanas may influence renal function and filtration rate. Research indicates that yoga practice can positively affect renal parameters, including glomerular filtration rate (GFR) and renal plasma flow (RPF). The mechanisms might entail enhanced vascular endothelial function, modulation of the autonomic nervous system, and decreased oxidative stress resulting from yogasana practice, potentially leading to improvements in renal physiology [29].

13. Impact of yogasana on the reproductive system

The reproductive system is crucial for human reproduction and overall health. Yogasanas have been recognized as a beneficial practice for women's reproductive health. Specific poses and relaxation techniques may help regulate menstrual cycles, alleviate menstrual pain, and reduce symptoms of premenstrual syndrome (PMS). Additionally, yoga can promote fertility and support women going through various stages of reproductive life. Yogasanas, pranayama, and meditation may have potential implications for male reproductive health. Some studies have shown that regular yoga practice can improve sperm quality, hormonal balance, and overall fertility. This may be due to reduced stress levels, enhanced blood flow to reproductive organs, and improved endocrine function to improve the functioning of the reproductive system [30, 31].

14. Conclusion

This chapter review provides a thorough examination of the profound effects of Yogasana on both the human body and mind. Empirical evidence strongly supports the notion that regular Yogasana practice yields a multitude of physiological, biomechanical, and psychological benefits. Its potential as a therapeutic intervention for enhancing overall well-being and mental health is compelling. However, to fully unlock its therapeutic potential, further research is necessary to uncover the underlying mechanisms and refine its application across diverse clinical contexts. Through continued investigation and refinement, Yogasana stands poised to revolutionize holistic health and wellness practices for generations to come.

Author details

Sobika Rao and Rameswar Pal*
Morarji Desai National Institute of Yoga, Ministry of Ayush, Government of India, New Delhi, India

*Address all correspondence to: physioramupal@gmail.com

References

[1] Goyandkar H. Commentator: Patanjali Yog Darshan with Hindi Interpretation. India: Gita Press Gorakhpur; 2007

[2] Dayanidy G, Dayanidy R, Bhavanani AB. Principles and Methods of Yoga Practices. India: ICYER; 2017

[3] Yoga Swami Svatmarama. Hatha Yoga Pradipika. Elsy Becherer ed. India: The Aquarian Press; 1992

[4] Kuvalayananda S. Asanas. India: Kaivalyadhama; 1993

[5] Mandal D, Ray U, Ghosh P. Differences in skeletal growth pattern of yoga practising adolescent girls: A cross-sectional study. Journal of Ayurveda Integrated Medicine. 2022;**13**(2):100550. DOI: 10.1016/j.jaim.2022.100550

[6] Mullerpatan RP, Agarwal BM, Shetty T, Nehete GR, Narasipura OS. Kinematics of Suryanamaskar using three-dimensional motion capture. International Journal of Yoga. 2019;**12**(2):124-131. DOI: 10.4103/ijoy.IJOY_26_18

[7] Kanjirathingal JP, Mullerpatan RP, Nehete G, Raghuram N. Effect of Yogasana intervention on standing balance performance among people with diabetic peripheral neuropathy: A pilot study. International Journal of Yoga. 2021;**14**(1):60-70. DOI: 10.4103/ijoy.IJOY_75_20

[8] Gandolfi MG, Zamparini F, Spinelli A, Prati C. Āsana for neck, shoulders, and wrists to prevent musculoskeletal disorders among dental professionals: In-office Yóga protocol. Journal of Functional and Morphology Kinesiology. 2023;**8**(1):26. DOI: 10.3390/jfmk8010026

[9] Chellaa R, Soumya MS, Inbaraj G, Nayar R, Saidha PK, Menezes VH, et al. Impact of hatha yoga on the airway resistances in healthy individuals and allergic rhinitis patients. Indian Journal of Otolaryngology Head and Neck Surgery. 2019;**71**(Suppl. 3):1748-1756. DOI: 10.1007/s12070-017-1098-1

[10] Sarma SA. Effect of Yogasana on circulatory & respiratory system. International Journal of Physiology, Nutrition and Physical Education. 2018;**3**(1):190-192

[11] Nagarathna R, Nagendra HR. Yoga for bronchial asthma: A controlled study. British Medical Journal (Clin Res Ed). 1985;**291**(6502):1077-1079. DOI: 10.1136/bmj.291.6502.1077

[12] Bernotiene G, Slapsinskaite A, Berškienė K, Daunoravičienė A, Vainoras A, Razón S. Yoga's effects on the cardiovascular system of healthy women: Implications for best practices. Alternative Therapies in Health and Medicine. 2020;**26**(5):18-26

[13] Cowen VS. Functional fitness improvements after a worksite-based yoga initiative. Journal of Bodywork and Movement Therapies. 2010;**14**(1):50-54. DOI: 10.1016/j.jbmt. 2009. 02. 006

[14] Christa E, Srivastava P, Chandran DS, Jaryal AK, Yadav RK, Roy A, et al. Effect of yoga based cardiac rehabilitation on blood pressure variability and Baroreflex sensitivity: RCT in patients post MI. Applied Psychophysiology and Biofeedback. 2023;**48**(1):1-15. DOI: 10.1007/s10484-022-09561-3

[15] Ray US, Sinha B, Tomer OS, Pathak A, Dasgupta T, Selvamurthy W. Aerobic capacity & perceived exertion

after practice of hatha yogic exercises. The Indian Journal of Medical Research. 2001;**114**:215-221

[16] Pal R, Saha M, Chatterjee A, Halder K, Tomer OS, Pathak A, et al. Anaerobic power, muscle strength and physiological changes in physically active men following yogic practice. Biomedical Human Kinetics. 2014;**5**:113-120. DOI: 10.2478/bhk-2013-0017

[17] Iyengar BKS, Evans JJ, Abrams D. Light on Life: The Yoga Journey to Wholeness, Inner Peace, and Ultimate Freedom. 1st ed. USA: Rodale Press; 2005

[18] Setia G, Ramanathan M, Bhavanani AB, Prabu BSM. Adjuvant yoga therapy for symptom management of functional dyspepsia: A case series. Journal of Ayurveda Integrated Medicine. 2023;**14**(3):100715. DOI: 10.1016/j.jaim.2023.100715

[19] Pal R, Singh SN, Chatterjee A, and Saha M. Age – Related changes on cardiovascular system, autonomic function and levels of BDNF of healthy active males: Role of yogic practice. 2014;**36**(4):9683. DOI: 10.1007/s11357-014-9683-7

[20] Swanson A. Science of Yoga Understanding the Anatomy and Physiology to Perfect your Practice. London: DK Publisher; 2019

[21] Shree Ganesh HR, Subramanya P, Rao MR, Udupa V. Role of yoga therapy in improving digestive health and quality of sleep in an elderly population: A randomized controlled trial. Journal of Bodywork and Movement Therapies. 2021;**27**:692-697. DOI: 10.1016/j.jbmt.2021.04.012

[22] Wilke E, Reindl W, Thomann PA, Ebert MP, Wuestenberg T, Thomann AK. Effects of yoga in inflammatory bowel diseases and on frequent IBD-associated extraintestinal symptoms like fatigue and depression. Complementary Therapies in Clinical Practice. 2021;**45**:101465. DOI: 10.1016/j.ctcp.2021.101465

[23] Streeter CC, Jensen JE, Perlmutter RM, Cabral HJ, Tian H, Terhune DB, et al. Yoga asana sessions increase brain GABA levels: A pilot study. Journal of Alternative and Complementary Medicine. 2007;**13**(4):419-426. DOI: 10.1089/acm.2007.6338

[24] Jayaram N, Varambally S, Behere RV, Venkatasubramanian G, Arasappa R, Christopher R, et al. Effect of yoga therapy on plasma oxytocin and facial emotion recognition deficits in patients of schizophrenia. Indian Journal of Psychiatry. 2013;**55**(Suppl. 3):S409-S413. DOI: 10.4103/0019-5545.116318

[25] Naveen GH, Thirthalli J, Rao MG, Varambally S, Christopher R, Gangadhar BN. Positive therapeutic and neurotropic effects of yoga in depression: A comparative study. Indian Journal of Psychiatry. 2013;**55**(Suppl. 3):S400-S404. DOI: 10.4103/0019-5545.116313

[26] Pascoe MC, Thompson DR, Ski CF. Yoga, mindfulness-based stress reduction and stress-related physiological measures: A meta-analysis. Psychoneuroendocrinology. 2017;**86**:152-168

[27] Ross A, Thomas S. The health benefits of yoga and exercise: A review of comparison studies. Journal of Alternative and Complementary Medicine. 2010;**16**(1):3-12. DOI: 10.1089/acm.2009.0044

[28] Nilkantham S, Majumdar V, Singh A. Scientific yoga module for hypothyroidism: A study protocol for tele-yoga RCT. Contemporary Clinical

Trials Communications. 2023;**33**:101157. DOI: 10.1016/j.conctc.2023.101157

[29] Bordman R, Meaney C, Telner D. The effects of hot yoga on kidney function: An observational pilot and feasibility study. International Journal of Yoga Therapy. 2022;**32**:1. DOI: 10.17761/2022-D-21-00001

[30] Jose A, Nayak S, Rajesh A, Kamath N, Nalini M. Impact of relaxation therapy on premenstrual symptoms: A systematic review. Journal of Education Health Promotion. 2022;**11**(1):401. DOI: 10.4103/jehp.jehp_586_22

[31] Patel V, Menezes H, Menezes C, Bouwer S, Bostick-Smith CA, Speelman DL. Regular mindful yoga practice as a method to improve androgen levels in women with polycystic ovary syndrome: A randomized, controlled trial. Journal of American Osteopathic Association. 2020;**120**:323-335. DOI: 10.7556/jaoa.2020.050

Chapter 3

Harnessing the Power of Yoga: Understanding an Ancient Healing Tradition from a Holistic Perspective

Fadi Kayale

Abstract

This chapter introduces a holistic perspective of the Yogic tradition. First we review the healing power of yoga through the Eastern tradition, highlighting the importance of yoga in maintaining the Chakra system and sustaining a healthy Chi flow. We then endorse the healing power of yoga through a Western medical lens and evidence-based empirical research and clinical trials.

Keywords: yoga, holistic healing, alternative medicine, holistic perspective, energy medicine

1. Introduction

The twenty-first century is plagued by many astonishing inventions and a breakthrough in global connectedness. Human consciousness is entangled in a transhumanistic timeline, leading to a new quantum leap with an unknown fate. This quantum jump continues to challenge our understanding of its root and the quantum genesis of its existence.

As I am working on this book chapter, I cannot ignore the fact that Apple is on the verge of launching Vision Pro [1], an innovative device that has the potential to revolutionize our world. Although this innovative tool offers a captivating virtual experience, it fails to cure cancer, heal autoimmune disorders, or elucidate the underlying complexities of schizophrenia symptoms and psychopathology.

Our society has embraced a rigid Western medical approach that relies solely on psychopharmacology as an ultimate healing method, disregarding any advancements or research in the emerging field of quantum and bioenergetic medicine.

This chapter aims to demonstrate the adoption of the Yogic Tradition as a holistic modality that promotes a comprehensive approach to healing the human body, integrating both Eastern and Western perspectives.

2. Understanding yoga through the eastern tradition

2.1 A brief overview of chi

To understand the Eastern medical perspective, we need to define key concepts that preside over its approach. Alternative medicine manipulates energy flow throughout a living system to heal both its structural and bioenergetic components.

Chi, or Prana in Sanskrit, is a vital life source that flows through all living beings. The flow of Chi through the meridians is essential for maintaining the normal functions of the human body. If we want to describe it using an analogy, the meridians are to the bioenergetic body as the lymphatic system to the physiological body [2].

There are five main basic functions of Chi [3]:

1. *Movement and circulation:* Chi plays a vital role in the flow and transport of essential bodily fluids like lymph and blood. It also transports subtle energies such as electromagnetic and photonic particles, in particular Chi or Prana.

2. *Thermal regulation:* Chi plays a vital role in maintaining the physical body's homeostasis at an optimal temperature that promotes and nurtures life.

3. *Immune Function:* Chi has an important role in modulating our immune defenses against external pathogens or internal autoimmune attacks.

4. *Manifestation of life:* The flow of Chi is the essence of life; it sustains the body's bioenergetic, electromagnetic, and physiological functions; thus impacting the healthy functioning of the Chakras (as detailed in the following section).

5. *Maintenance of the Zang-fu organs:* In traditional Chinese medicine (TCM), maintaining the optimal functioning of the Zang-fu organs relies on the flow of Chi. The Zang-fu organs include the heart, liver, spleen, lung, kidneys, and the stomach.

At times, the flow of Chi to the internal organs and bioenergetic centers becomes obstructed. Factors include traumatic life events, emotional stress, synthetic medications, and drug abuse.

The accumulation of excessive bodily fluids such as lymph and blood after surgeries can also obstruct the flow of Chi. That is why surgeons advise patients to rest and practice self-care until total remission so that the accumulated fluids can totally dissipate [4].

Now that we have a basic understanding of Chi, let us delve into how this vital energy maintains the harmonious balance of our major energy centers, commonly known as the Chakras.

2.2 The relationship between the chakras and chi

In the human body, each cluster of organs translates energetically into an energetic center called Chakra. The flow of Chi into those energy centers maintains their normal functioning [5]. To further understand the role of Chi in those energy centers, let us briefly introduce them (**Figure 1**).

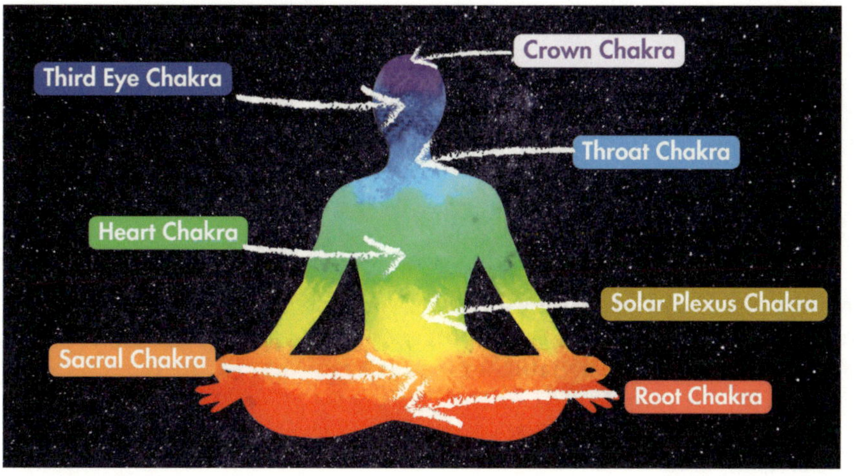

Figure 1.
The seven chakras of the human body.

2.2.1 The root chakra

The root Chakra is located at the base of the spine. It holds the large intestine, kidneys, bladder, rectum, sciatic nerve, bottom of the feet, and the adrenal glands. The photonic signature of this Chakra is red and shelters our human identity, stability, and grounding [6].

2.2.2 The sacral chakra

The sacral Chakra is located below the belly button. The organs within this area include the stomach, upper intestines, liver, gallbladder, spleen, kidneys, pancreas, reproductive organs, adrenal glands, middle spine, and the body's immune system. The photonic signature of this Chakra is orange and arouses our human sexuality, pleasure, and creativity centers [7].

2.2.3 The solar plexus

The Solar Plexus is located in the upper abdomen, precisely above the belly button. This specific energy center is closely connected to the celiac plexus and plays a crucial role in the regulation of the sympathetic nervous system. The photonic signature of this Chakra is yellow and represents our self-esteem, confidence, reality manifestation, protection, and growth [8].

2.2.4 The heart chakra

The heart Chakra is located at the center of the chest. The physiologic responsibility of the heart Chakra lies in the proper functioning of the heart, lungs and circulatory system. The photonic signature of this Chakra is green; it houses and evokes our human compassion and empathy toward one another [9].

2.2.5 The throat chakra

The throat Chakra is located within the throat region. This particular Chakra plays an important role in regulating the energetic flow through the thyroid gland. The photonic signature of this Chakra is light blue and accommodates the skills of communication and verbal power [10].

2.2.6 The third eye

The third eye, or the Ajna, is located between the eyes on the forehead. In our physical body, it corresponds to the hypothalamus, the pituitary gland, the eyes, ears, and the nose. The photonic signature of the Ajna is indigo and includes the gifts of intuition and imagination [11].

2.2.7 The crown chakra

The crown Chakra is located at the top of the head. This Chakra regulates the flow of Chi through the pituitary gland, the pineal gland, and the hypothalamus. The crown's photonic signature emanates a brilliant violet hue. This particular Chakra connects us to our higher states of consciousness, enlightenment, universal intelligence, and spirituality [12].

The Chakra centers are nurtured by a continuous flow of Chi. This flow energizes the cluster of organs that each Chakra harbors. When the Chi flow is blocked in any of the major Chakra centers, it can lead to imbalances, illness, and potentially fatal consequences [13].

Along with acupuncture, Ayurveda, Qigong, tai chi, and many other Eastern traditions, yoga plays an important role in harmonizing and balancing the Chi flow [14].

2.3 Understanding how yoga balances the flow of chi

Yoga is a mind-body technique that involves the mindful practice of posture, meditation, and breathing. This combination is renowned for its ability to harmonize the Chakras while promoting a healthy flow of Chi to essential organs [15].

Hatha yoga, an influential yoga discipline, emphasizes the removal of Chi blockages and the initiation of the healing process through the integration of postures, meditative states, and controlled breathing concomitantly during the practice of various postures and movements [16].

2.4 The practice of yoga is based on four important principles

The first principle dictates that the human body is a complex and interconnected system, encompassing various dimensions related to its structural, physiological, and bioenergetic aspects. Any disruption in one of those dimensions can have a detrimental effect on the overall well-being of a living entity, leading to an imbalance in the body's normal functions. The second principle states that each human is unique, and this uniqueness needs to be celebrated and respected. The third principle stresses that yoga is an empowering technique that pushes the student to be an intrinsic part of his healing process. The fourth principle of yoga states that the power of the mindset is crucial during the healing process. A positive mindset accelerates the healing process and the capacity to master yoga techniques in shorter terms [17].

Having grasped the connection between Chi, human physiology, and the Chakra system, as well as how yoga aids in eliminating blockages and fostering the healing process, let us now delve into the Western perspective.

3. Yoga through a Western lens

3.1 Introduction

In the previous sections, we have viewed a brief explanation of yoga's mechanism of action for healing the body and promoting well-being. Traditional Chinese medicine and the Hindu tradition both perceive this practice as a holistic modality that has an impact on our anatomy, physiology, and consciousness.

Despite skepticism among Western practitioners, extensive research provides compelling evidence of the numerous benefits of yoga and its profound impact on our physiology. In the following sections, we will investigate some scientific discoveries that endorse the Eastern perspective's claims regarding the healing power of yoga.

3.2 The physiologic effects of yoga

During prehistoric times, our ancestors could not have survived if intrinsic autonomic nervous activations did not exist. These evolutionary mechanisms are governed by our autonomic nervous system (ANS). Under circumstances that require attention and alertness, the autonomic nervous system activates the sympathetic nervous system, which is responsible for "fight or flight" responses such as increased alertness, energy, heart rate, and perspiration [18]. Moreover, when we require a moment to unwind, particularly following a substantial meal, our autonomic nervous system triggers the parasympathetic nervous system [19]. This system facilitates the "rest and digest" reactions, including relaxation, salivation, and a reduction in heart rate (**Figure 2**) [20].

Practicing yoga promotes relaxation, slow breathing, and mindfulness, with a deep focus on current posture and the present moment. By varying these maneuvers in various ways throughout a session, the parasympathetic system gets stimulated, inducing a peaceful and rejuvenating physiological state. Neuroscientists have discovered that yoga effectively suppresses the activity of the sympathetic area of the hypothalamus, leading to optimized responses to stress and a balanced parasympathetic system in the body. Yoga also seems to modulate the vagus nerve's activity, one of the main nerves of the parasympathetic nervous system. A groundbreaking study revealed that after just 1 month of yoga practice, there was a significant increase in vagal nerve activity, indicating enhanced parasympathetic nervous system responses. Additionally, yoga appears to suppress brain regions associated with aggressiveness, rage, and fear while stimulating median forebrain regions that are renowned for promoting a state of bliss. Several studies have demonstrated that this particular inhibition resulted in reduced anxiety, heart rate, respiratory rate, blood pressure, and cardiac output in individuals who engaged in yoga [21].

Yoga poses also have a remarkable ability to regulate and harmonize our circulatory system. Twisting poses, for example, create compression on venous blood within the internal organs. This compression leads to a surge of oxygenated blood flow when the pressure is released. This boosts blood circulation and hemoglobin levels, leading to increased oxygen delivery to the cells, thereby improving their function [22].

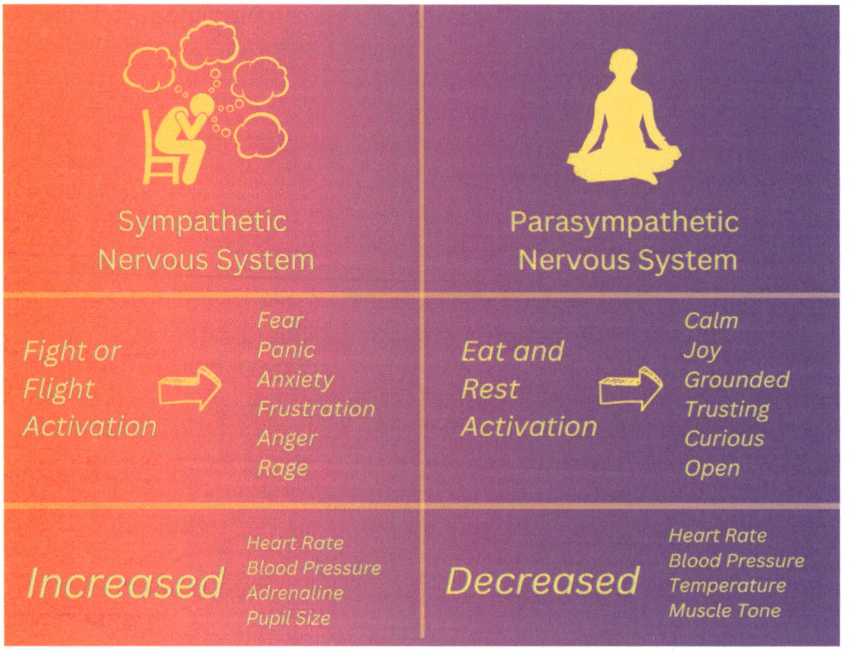

Figure 2.
The autonomic nervous system.

Moreover, several studies have shown that monitoring the hemodynamics of individuals who practice yoga has led to impressive benefits, such as lower resting heart rates, increased stamina, and improved utilization of oxygen during physical exertion [23]. As a result, these findings suggest that yoga has the potential to greatly enhance cardiovascular function and dramatically decrease the risk of heart attacks [24].

3.3 The effects of yoga on oxidative stress

The cells of the human body generate harmful molecules called free radicals. Those molecules are the underlying etiology of many neurodegenerative, autoimmune, and inflammatory diseases. The body scavenges those molecules with the help of another family of molecules called antioxidants. The latter can be either produced intrinsically or simply supplemented through a healthy diet [25]. Oxidative stress occurs when an imbalance between the production and the scavenging of free radicals takes place (**Figure 3**) [26].

There could be various factors contributing to this mechanism, including a lack of essential vitamins, a compromised immune system, and high levels of stress due to adverse life events [27].

A generous amount of research studies demonstrated that yoga impacts the body's levels of oxidative stress. In one particular study, researchers discovered that individuals who practiced yoga for over 2 years experienced significantly reduced levels of oxidative stress in their bodies. These findings highlight the incredible long-term benefits that yoga can have on our overall well-being [28]. There is preliminary speculation that yoga indeed plays a major role in lowering physiological cortisol levels and inflammatory markers [29].

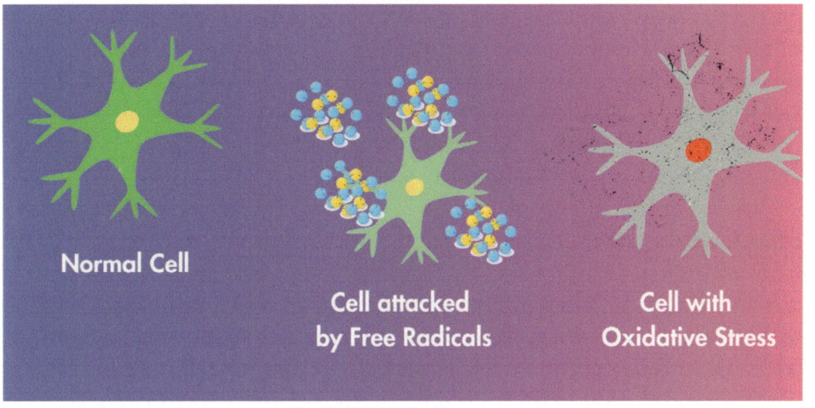

Figure 3.
A brief overview of oxidative stress.

In conclusion, practicing yoga seems to reduce cortisol levels, thereby modifying the processes that lead to increased levels of free radicals and inflammation [30].

3.4 The effects of yoga on cognitive functions

There has been extensive research examining the relationship between yoga and its impact on cognitive functions. In particular, one study compared differences in cortical thickness among practitioners of Hatha yoga. Yoga practitioners showed a significant increase in the volume of their hippocampus, a region of the brain that plays a key role in memory, as previously discovered by neuroscientists [31].

The results of that study also showed a clear change in electroencephalogram (EEG) brainwaves, with a decrease in delta waves and an increase in alpha, theta, and beta brainwaves. This compelling evidence indicates a considerable enhancement in memory, concentration, and overall synchronization of brain activity [32]. Another clinical trial suggested that the improvement of cognitive functions is proportional to the years of practice of yoga, suggesting the added value of long-term regular practice [33].

Yoga improves the brain's functional connectivity, which normally decreases with age [34]. This indicates that yoga has a crucial role in slowing down cognitive decline. Furthermore, yoga can enhance the circulation of blood to various areas of the brain, including the prefrontal cortex and frontal lobes, making it a promising potential intervention among individuals who previously had a stroke [35].

3.5 The effect of yoga on cancer

Cancer patients are faced with an everlasting effect of stress emanating both from chemotherapy treatment and the disease itself. Yoga, breathing exercises, and mindfulness altogether seem to improve the quality of life of individuals diagnosed with cancer.

Multiple research studies have shown that yoga helps invigorate patients' mental and physical energy by reducing fatigue.

Similar to mindfulness practice, yoga can help patients to stay grounded in the present moment without feeling consumed by the prognosis of their condition or treatment outcomes [36].

One particular study showed that yoga can reduce post-chemotherapy-related side effects such as toxicity, nausea, and fatigue [37]. Restorative postures, savasana, pranayama, and meditation encourage pratyahara, a turning inward of the senses that enable downtime for the nervous system, the byproduct often being improved sleep [38]. On the other hand, further research is required to investigate the effects of yoga practice on the physiology of this specific group [39].

3.6 The effects of yoga on mental health

Yoga seems to play an important role in alleviating the symptoms of various mental health disorders. For example, yoga tends to reduce both post-traumatic stress disorder (PTSD) and depression symptoms among diagnosed women [40]. Recent research demonstrated that practicing yoga leads to a significant reduction in the symptoms of anxiety disorders and panic attacks [41].

Moreover, a combination of yoga and cognitive behavioral therapy (CBT) seems to play an important role in alleviating the symptoms of panic disorder [24]. Similarly, other studies explored the effect of yoga on depression. The consensus is that the combination of yoga and antidepressant as a holistic intervention was superior to solely prescribing antidepressants as a pharmacological first-line treatment [42].

3.7 The effects of yoga on neurodegenerative and inflammatory disease

There is extensive scientific literature related to the positive effects of yoga on neurodegenerative and inflammatory diseases. In multiple sclerosis, a single-arm study demonstrated that the practice of yoga can improve balance and walking speed. Additional research showed that yoga also enhances the patient's quality of life and diminishes associated symptoms of chronic fatigue [43].

Recent research also revealed the benefits of yoga among patients diagnosed with chronic fatigue syndrome [44]. The latter's clinical presentation is a complex combination of symptoms such as fatigue, insomnia, sensitivity to light, difficulty concentrating, and chronic headaches.

Similarly. yoga has a positive effect on alleviating symptoms of inflammatory diseases. Yoga appears to reduce pain, inflammation, and stiffness among patients diagnosed with rheumatoid arthritis [45].

Due to the chapter's limited scope, it is worth noting that numerous research studies have also demonstrated the positive healing effect of yoga on a wide range of other conditions, such as asthma, COPD, and low back pain [46].

4. Conclusion

In this chapter, we introduced the Eastern and Western perspectives regarding the practice of yoga. In the Eastern tradition, yoga, Chi flow, and the Chakra system are all interconnected. The three systems work harmoniously together, and an imbalance in one of them can seriously inflict damage to the physical and etheric body. Empirical research allowed the Western perspective to believe in the healing power of the Yogic tradition equally. This opens the door to further expanding the scope of research and clinical trials to other available alternative healing modalities such as acupuncture, herbal medicine, cupping, and more.

Author details

Fadi Kayale
The University of Toronto, Canada

*Address all correspondence to: fa.kayale@mail.utoronto.ca

References

[1] Liao W, Dang C, Pan W. The brief theory of viscus and its manifestations in traditional Chinese medicine. Integrative Medicine International. 2017;**4**(1-2):13-18

[2] Leffer L. What Apple's New Vision Pro Headset Might Do to Our Brain. New York, NY: Scientific American; 2024 [Internet]. Available from: https://www.scientificamerican.com/article/what-apples-new-vision-pro-headset-might-do-to-our-brain/ [Accessed: March 2, 2024]

[3] Kirkham D. In: Kirkham D, DAOM, EAMP, LAC, editors. What is Qi? Flow & Traffic Jams on the Qi Superhighway [Internet]. Washington; 2016. Available from: https://acupuncturistseattle.com/what-qi-chi-health/ [Accessed: March 2, 2024]

[4] Stanley-Baker M, Qi 氣. Routledge Handbook of Chinese Medicine. [Internet]. London: Routledge; 2022. pp. 23-50. DOI: 10.4324/9780203740262-4 [Accessed: March 2, 2024]

[5] Heilijgers-Seelen DM. The System of Five Cakras in Kubjikāmatatantra 14-16. Leiden, The Netherlands: Brill; 1994

[6] Lopez C. Review of: The Devī Gītā: The song of the goddess: A translation, annotation, and commentary. By C. Mackenzie Brown. Albany: State University of New York Press, 1998. Journal of Asian Studies. 2002;**61**(1):289-290

[7] A concise dictionary of Indian philosophy [Internet]. Available from: https://books.google.com/books?id=qcoUFYOX0bEC

[8] Richards G, Bernard T. Hindu philosophy. Religious Studies. 1983;**19**(4):544-544

[9] Beshara R. The chakra system as a bio-socio-psycho-spiritual model of consciousness: Anahata: As heart-centered consciousness. Journal of Applied Consciousness Studies. 1 Jan 2013;**1**(1):29-33

[10] Mageau M. They Come in Peace and Love. 2014

[11] Baker D. The Third Eye. Wisconsin, USA: New Leaf Distribution Company; 1981

[12] Simpson L. The Book of Chakra Healing. Sterling Publishing Company, Inc.; 1999

[13] Selby A. The Chakra Energy Plan: The Practical 7-Step Program to Balance and Revitalize. Independence, OH: Sterling Publishing Company; 2006

[14] Singh Khalsa SB. Kundalini yoga and kundalini awakenings. Complementary Therapies in Clinical Practice. 2022;**47**:101417

[15] Ivanhoe PJ, Norden BWV. Readings in Classical Chinese Philosophy. Indianapolis, IN, USA: Hackett Publishing Company; 2023

[16] Bernard T. Hatha Yoga: The Report of a Personal Experience. New York, NY, USA: Columbia University Press; 1955

[17] Feuerstein G. The Path of Yoga: An Essential Guide to its Principles and Practices. Boulder, Colorado: Shambhala Publications; 2011

[18] Nilsson S, Holmgren S. Comparative Physiology and Evolution of the Autonomic Nervous System [Internet]. London: Routledge; 2021. DOI: 10.1201/9781315139807 [Accessed: March 2, 2024]

[19] Langley JN. The Autonomic Nervous System. Cambridge, UK: Cambridge University Press; 1921

[20] Koeppen BM, Stanton BA, Hall JM, Swiatecka-Urban A. Berne & Levy Physiology. 8th ed. Philadelphia, PA: Elsevier; 2023. pp. 218-230

[21] Field T. Yoga research review. Complementary Therapies in Clinical Practice. 2016;**24**:145-161

[22] Yunati M, Deshpande V, Yuwanate A. Dynamics of heart rate induced by Sahaja yoga meditation in healthy normal subjects above 40 years. National Journal of Physiology, Pharmacy and Pharmacology. 2014;**4**(1):80

[23] Sharma SK. Effect of selected asanas in hatha yoga on muscular endurance, flexibility and vital capacity among yoga students. International Journal of Physical Education Sports Management and Yogic Sciences. 2022;**12**(2):42-47

[24] Harinath K, Malhotra AS, Pal K, Prasad R, Kumar R, Kain TC, et al. Effects of hatha yoga and Omkar meditation on cardiorespiratory performance, psychologic profile, and melatonin secretion. The Journal of Alternative and Complementary Medicine. 2004;**10**(2):261-268

[25] Preedy VR, Watson RR. Handbook of Disease Burdens and Quality of Life Measures. New York, NY: Springer New York; 2010. pp. 4278-4280

[26] Birnboim HC. Importance of DNA Strand-Break Damage in Tumor Promotion. Atomic Energy of Canada Limited; 1983

[27] Lennon SV, Martin SJ, Cotter TG. Dose-dependent induction of apoptosis in human tumour cell lines by widely diverging stimuli. Cell Proliferation. 1991;**24**(2):203-214

[28] Krishna BH, Keerthi GS, Kumar CK, Reddy NM. Association of leukocyte telomere length with oxidative stress in yoga practitioners. Journal of Clinical and Diagnostic Research. 2015;**9**(3):CC01-CC03. DOI: 10.7860/JCDR/2015/13076.5729

[29] Riley KE, Park CL. How does yoga reduce stress? A systematic review of mechanisms of change and guide to future inquiry. Health Psychology Review. 2015;**9**(3):379-396

[30] Butzer B, Day D, Potts A, Ryan C, Coulombe S, Davies B, et al. Effects of a classroom-based yoga intervention on cortisol and behavior in second- and third-grade students. Journal of Evidence-Based Complementary & Alternative Medicine. 2014;**20**(1):41-49

[31] Gothe NP, McAuley E. Yoga and cognition. Psychosomatic Medicine. 2015;77(7):784-797

[32] Desai R, Tailor A, Bhatt T. Effects of yoga on brain waves and structural activation: A review. Complementary Therapies in Clinical Practice. 2015;**21**(2):112-118

[33] Villemure C, Čeko M, Cotton VA, Bushnell MC. Neuroprotective effects of yoga practice: Age-, experience-, and frequency-dependent plasticity. Frontiers in Human Neuroscience. 12 May 2015;**9**:281. DOI: 10.3389/fnhum.2015.00281

[34] Gaskins R, Jennings E, Thind H, Becker B, Bock B. Acute and cumulative effects of Vinyasa yoga on affect and stress among college students participating in an eight-week yoga program: A pilot study. International Journal of Yoga Therapy. 2014;**24**(1):63-70

[35] Gothe NP, Khan I, Hayes J, Erlenbach E, Damoiseaux JS. Yoga effects

on brain health: A systematic review of the current literature. Brain Plasticity. 2019;**5**(1):105-122

[36] Wurz A, Chamorro-Vina C, Guilcher GMT, Schulte F, Culos-Reed SN. The feasibility and benefits of a 12-week yoga intervention for pediatric cancer out-patients. Pediatric Blood & Cancer. 2014;**61**(10):1828-1834

[37] Carson JW, Carson KM, Porter LS, Keefe FJ, Shaw H, Miller JM. Yoga for women with metastatic breast cancer: Results from a pilot study. Journal of Pain and Symptom Management. 2007;**33**(3):331-341

[38] McCall MC, Ward A, Heneghan C. Yoga in adult cancer: A pilot survey of attitudes and beliefs among oncologists. Current Oncology. 2015;**22**(1):13-19

[39] Sharma P, Sampliner R. Barrett's Esophagus and Esophageal Adenocarcinoma. Hoboken, New Jersey: John Wiley & Sons; 2008

[40] Jindani F, Turner N, Khalsa SBS. A yoga intervention for posttraumatic stress: A preliminary randomized control trial. Evidence-Based Complementary and Alternative Medicine. 2015;**2015**:1-8

[41] Johnston JM, Minami T, Greenwald D, Li C, Reinhardt K, Khalsa SBS. Yoga for military service personnel with PTSD: A single arm study. Psychological Trauma: Theory, Research, Practice, and Policy. 2015;7(6):555-562

[42] Sheffield KM, Woods-Giscombé CL. Efficacy, feasibility, and acceptability of perinatal yoga on Women's mental health and well-being. Journal of Holistic Nursing. 2015;**34**(1):64-79

[43] Guner S, Inanici F. Yoga therapy and ambulatory multiple sclerosis assessment of gait analysis parameters, fatigue and balance. Journal of Bodywork and Movement Therapies. 2015;**19**(1):72-81

[44] Oka T, Tanahashi T, Chijiwa T, Lkhagvasuren B, Sudo N, Oka K. Isometric yoga improves the fatigue and pain of patients with chronic fatigue syndrome who are resistant to conventional therapy: A randomized, controlled trial. BioPsychoSocial Medicine. Dec 2014;**8**:1-9

[45] Moonaz SH, Bingham CO III, Wissow L, Bartlett SJ. Yoga in sedentary adults with arthritis: Effects of a randomized controlled pragmatic trial. The Journal of Rheumatology. 2015;**42**(7):1194-1202

[46] Ross A, Thomas S. The health benefits of yoga and exercise: A review of comparison studies. The Journal of Alternative and Complementary Medicine. 2010;**16**(1):3-12

Chapter 4

Yoga-nidrā: A State of Mind, *Not* a Technique

Stephen Parker

Abstract

Since its introduction to the West in 1969 by Swāmī Rāma through experiments conducted at the U.S. Menninger Foundation, *yoga-nidrā* has become a popular practice among yoga teachers from many traditions. The result is a patchwork of techniques incorporating a variety of practices and procedures. It has come to be thought of primarily as technique and the variability of techniques across traditions has engendered debate about which technique is right. In fact, *yoga-nidrā* is defined by Swāmī Rāma, as well as by textual sources, as a state of mind where the practitioner consciously enters a state of deep, dreamless (non-REM) sleep, remaining both inwardly aware and aware of their external surroundings. The more a practitioner has managed to keep the parasympathetic relaxation system continuously activated through moment-to-moment mindfulness practice, the less technique is required to enter that state. The only way to be certain that someone has entered this state is to measure their brain waves with an electro-encephalogram (EEG) for predominance of delta waves and to test their awareness of their surroundings. For purposes of getting to the state of *yoga-nidrā*, any of the preparatory techniques will serve, although none are a guarantee that the state will be reached.

Keywords: *yoga-nidrā*, mindfulness, sleep, relaxation, brain waves

1. Introduction

Swāmī Rāma of the Himālayas first appeared in the United States in 1969. One of his hosts, Daniel Ferguson M.D., connected him to the Voluntary Controls Project of Drs. Elmer and Alyce Green at the Menninger Foundation, a psychiatric research institution that had begun to investigate mind–body interactions [1] Swāmī Rāma's intention was to demonstrate to people in the West what a human being can achieve through the kind of mental mastery provided by yoga. As part of this project, he agreed to demonstrate all of the different brain wave states. At this time there was great interest in alpha-wave states as a way to use technology to help people induce deep relaxation. He not only demonstrated alpha-wave states, but went on to demonstrate theta- and delta-wave states as well, something that the science of the time hardly thought possible through conscious effort. In the demonstration of the delta-wave state (deep, dreamless sleep), his brain waves were monitored by an electroencephalogram (EEG). Most surprising was that, during the experiment, two lab technicians were having a conversation nearby, and when Swāmī Rāma came out of the *yoga-nidrā* state, he was able to recount their conversation word-for-word. In that experiment he used no technique to enter that mental state. When he taught *yoga-nidrā* publically, however, he taught a series of relaxation practices as necessary preliminaries for people who had not otherwise learned to keep their minds continually still, clear, relaxed and aware [2].

One of Swāmī Rāma's more advanced disciples, Swāmī Veda Bhāratī, formerly Dr. Uṣarbudh Ārya, endeavored in 2006 to replicate that experiment in the laboratory of Dean Radin Ph.D. at the Institute for Noetic Sciences in Petaluma, CA [3]. As Radin recounts, he realized as they were talking before the formal experiment, that the EEG was already running and Swāmī Veda was producing almost pure delta waves as they talked! This was extraordinary as neuroscience would predict that the delta-wave state is one where the subject remains unconscious as all the neurons in their nervous system fire synchronously. This persuaded Radin that it was very likely that Swāmī Veda remained in a state of *yoga-nidrā* most or all of the time, waking or sleeping (p. 69). As a result of his training by Swāmī Rāma, Swāmī Veda recognized that he had been using states of *yoga-nidrā* without knowing what they were since early childhood [4]. Later in life, he would often pause in the midst of a lecture ("just give me a minute") to use *yoga-nidrā* to stave off a cardiac crisis. In some form, this would occur daily during the last 20 years or so of his bodily life. (He once told the author that since his open heart surgery in 1992, he had not been without angina, cardiac heart pain, for one second.) Though cardiac pain was always present, he rarely showed it and remained joyful and even-minded to the public eye.

2. Swāmī Veda Bhāratī's model for levels of practice

For a conference on *yoga-nidrā* in 2009, Swāmī Veda suggested a model for *yoga-nidrā* practice which had four levels ([5], pp. 11–12), described both experientially and with testable physiological hypotheses:

1. The first level comprises preparatory deep relaxation. It is characterized by a predominance of alpha waves measured via electroencephalography (8–13 Hz). Here one may accomplish significant psychophysiological changes including reduction of blood pressure and migraine headaches. This level is very similar to the states attained in clinical hypnosis. This author suspects that clinical hypnosis is a special case of *yoga-nidrā*.

2. The second level is characterized by a predominance of theta waves (4–8 Hz), verging on delta waves (0.5–4 Hz) at deeper levels of practice. This is the level at which one may work with creativity, making decisions, exercising intentions (*saṁkalpa*), doing invention and composition. This author observed Swāmī Veda dictating his commentary on the *Yoga-sūtras of Patañjali* from that state, which was his preferred process of writing.

3. In level three, the preparatory practices bring the practitioner to the state of *yoga-nidrā* proper. In the beginning there may be theta waves which eventually gives way to a predominance of delta waves (0.5–4 Hz) and the experience of observing deep, non-REM (rapid eye movement) sleep with both inner and outer awareness, from an inner cave in the heart center, *anāhata-cakra*. This is

the experience of *abhāva-pratyaya* described in *Yoga-sūtras* I.10 [6]. Entering this state may require direct induction through a process of initiation by a qualified teacher.

4. Progression to level four requires mastery of the first three levels, meaning that the person can enter the state of *yoga-nidrā* with no technique and no preliminaries. This stage has no time limits. Practitioners often remain in this state up to 3.5 hours, the balance of his/her sleep taken in the ordinary manner. Mastery of all four levels brings the practitioner to the doorstep of *turīya*. Contrary to the claims of some teachers, Swāmī Veda always clearly explained that *yoga-nidrā* is not equivalent to *turīya*.

3. Research investigation of *yoga-nidrā*

In 2012 the author undertook an effort to assess the quality of scientific research on *yoga-nidrā* since it seemed to hold so much promise as a support to peoples' physical and mental health and it provided testable hypotheses [5, 7, 8]. At that time there were only a very few published studies that measured subjects' brain waves in order to ascertain whether the preparatory techniques utilized actually brought the subjects to the state of *yoga-nidrā*. Without this instrumentation, it really is not possible to objectively assess the effectiveness of any of the preparatory practices. These studies all demonstrated that subjects got deeply relaxed, but that is not hard to show through questionnaires, electromyography or measures of pulse or blood pressure, and this much has been done many times over. In the past several years, the experimental methodologies have begun to utilize brain wave measurement and other more rigorous methods (e.g. full polysomnographic sleep studies) and so the author has high hopes that this will provide significant results [9, 10]. In the studies cited, it already has.

4. Textual descriptions

The textual descriptions of *yoga-nidrā* are several and mention of *yoga-nidrā* dates from as early as the early Upaniṣads to the relatively late texts of *haṭhayoga* and systematic *advaita-vedānta*. The paucity of detail in the early texts can be attributed to the fact that the practice was taught master-to-disciple from the oral-initiatory tradition of yoga because the technique was always customized to the particular needs and abilities of the disciple ([11], pp. 786–811). In *Bhagavad-gītā* II.69, there is the cryptic verse about how yogis remain aware in what is night for ordinary beings and ordinary beings are active during what is night (= unconscious, habit-based living) to the yogis. Arjuna is also often referred to by Kṛṣṇa as *Guḍakeṣa*, "master of sleep," one of the pre-requisites for the initiation he is given in chapter 11. The state of *yoga-nidrā* is described in several sources. Couture (1999) focuses primarily on the mythical literature in the *Mahābhārata* and *Purāṇas*. Parker et al. ([5], p. 13) and Pandi-Perumal et al. ([9], pp. 84–85) also utilize descriptions from the *Yogatarāvali* of *Śaṅkarācārya*, the *Haṭhayogapradīpikā* and *Śāṇḍilya-upaniṣad*. These later sources give a somewhat more detailed practical description of *yoga-nidrā*.

To summarize these descriptions, all three of these sources focus on activation of the *suṣumnā-ṇāḍī*, where the ordinary alternation of activity in the right and left nostrils is transcended and both nostrils remain equally open, indicating simultaneous activation of both cerebral hemispheres. The practitioner enters a state of *unmani* ("upward mind") which, when extended, becomes *yoga-nidrā.* Some interpreters claim that this is a form of *pratyāhāra*, sensory withdrawal. This, however, is not the case as one of the features of *yoga-nidrā* demonstrated by Swāmī Rāma, is that the practitioner retains awareness of his/her surroundings. In *pratyāhāra*, the senses are entirely withdrawn from their external surroundings and sense objects and dissolve completely back into *manas* (*Yoga-sūtra* II.54) [11]. These texts also state that the activity of *manas*, the lower, sensory and thinking mind, ceases altogether. In other words, the lower sensory mind goes to sleep while the higher mind, *buddhi*, observes the process.

Śaṅkarācārya's Yogatarāvali also encourages the practitioner to remain in a state of *turīya*. This has prompted some teachers to maintain that *yoga-nidrā* is *turīya* itself, the fourth state of consciousness in the Advaita system, or that it is a state of *samādhi*. Swāmī Veda often cautioned that neither of these is true. *Turīya* in particular, he said, is the process of *nirvikalpa-* or *asamprajñāta-samādhi* infusing permanently into all other states of consciousness like oil spreading over the surface of water. In his descriptions of these inner states, Swāmī Rāma explained that *yoga-nidrā* brings one very close to *samādhi*, since deep sleep and *samādhi* are very similar, *samādhi* being conscious and deep sleep being, usually, unconscious. *Yoga-nidrā* gradually wears away the boundary between them so that, as Lakshmanjoo explains, based on *Kṣemarāja*'s commentary on *Śiva-sutras* I.11 ([12], pp. 39–44), most people's first experience of *samādhi* occurs in sleep rather than in meditation.

5. Technique and preparation for *yoga-nidrā*

The "technique" for *yoga-nidrā* itself is quite simple: from the activated *suṣumnā-ṇāḍī*, sink your awareness into a silent cave in the heart (*anāhata*) cakra with no thought and only the awareness of breath/*prāṇa*. Most people cannot achieve the required absence of distracting thoughts as a result of unresolved emotional conflicts that tend to be carried in their bodily tissues, their mind and their relationships. For them, it requires an effort to totally relax each layer (*koṣa*) of the body–mind: physical body (*anna-maya*), energy body (*prāṇa-maya*), lower mental/sensory body (*mano-*maya) and the higher mental body (*vijñāna-maya*). Hence the array of preparatory practices of various traditions [13–15]. It is important not to confuse these preparatory practices for the state of *yoga-nidrā* and, similarly, to confuse verbally facilitated relaxation with *yoga-nidrā*. The lifetime process of making the body–mind clear, pleasant and stable so that the body–mind can remain perpetually relaxed and concentrated is referred to by Patañjali (I.33) as *citta-prasādana*, "making the mind-field clear, pleasant and stable" [6]. This is the principal subject of the external limbs of yoga practice which prepare the body–mind to enter (and remain in) deep states of meditation [16].

So, for most people, a series of relaxation practices are necessary to accomplish this multi-level, preparatory relaxation. All of these various methods can work and none of them are a guarantee of reaching the state of *yoga-nidrā*. There is no way to compare the methods empirically because their success depends to a large degree on the quality of steady state relaxation of the subjects. The generic method taught by Swāmī Rāma ([2], pp. 186–191) for a general audience involves the following and takes this author about 90 min to complete when leading it with a group:

1. General progressive muscle relaxation. The more points of concentration, the deeper the relaxation is likely to be.

2. 61-point relaxation, often referred to as *śavayātra*, "the pilgrimage through the corpse," where 61 *marma* points are visualized going through the body.

3. *Śithali-karaṇa*, a practice where breath/*prāṇa* is visualized sweeping down the body with exhalation and up the body with inhalation, stopping the flow at the toes (10 times), then the ankles (10 times), then the knees (10 times), then the perineum (5 times), then the navel center (5 times), then the heart center (5 times), then the throat center (5 times), then between the eyebrow center and the spot where the nosebridge meets the upper lip (5 times), then from the crown of the head to the eyebrow center (5 times) and then down the body from crown to throat center, crown to heart center and so forth in reverse order, down to the toes.

4. Five breaths through the eyebrow center (controls the waking state), five breaths through the throat center (controls he dream state) and five breaths through the heart center (controls deep sleep).

5. Then awareness is taken into the heart center cave with no thought other than the awareness of breath. Remain for up to 10 minutes and then exit gently and gradually, maintaining breath awareness. This limitation of ten minutes was never directly explained by Swāmī Rāma. According to Swāmī Veda Bhāratī ([3], p. 61), practicing longer than ten minutes conditions the mind to states that are in the sub-delta range of brain waves, 0–0.5 Hz, a coma-like state which is the *bhava-pratyaya* state described in *Yoga-sutra* I.19, which, contrary to some interpreters of the *sutra*, is not a high state of *samādhi*.

Swāmī Veda taught a number of abbreviated methods designed for those with deeper steady-state relaxation, none of which have been published. He taught these on an individual basis. Other teachers have assembled differing sets of preparatory practices, the most popular of which are the ones propounded by Swāmī Satyānanda Saraswatī of the Bihar School of Yoga [13–15] Once again, any of these sets of preliminaries can prepare a practitioner to enter *yoga-nidrā*, although none of them is a guarantee of reaching that state.

6. Health benefits of *yoga-nidrā*

The health benefits of *yoga-nidrā* generally parallel the many benefits of ordinary sleep. Sleep science has demonstrated that across almost all disease categories, sleep has the largest overall positive effect size as a therapy [17]. Most of these cluster around strengthening a person's parasympathetic relaxation system, the rest, relax and restore system. Modern life easily exploits the vigilant bias of our nervous system towards the need to respond quickly to threats via the largely sympathetic autonomic stress response systems (so-called "fight, flee or freeze"). *Yoga-nidrā* greatly strengthens a person's ability to maintain steady-state relaxation.

Pandi-Perumal et al. [9] have reviewed the empirical studies of therapeutic benefits in some detail. This is a summary of their review:

Several studies demonstrated significant improvement in the ability to maintain a state of relaxation along with significant reductions in mild to moderate anxiety and depression. This was measured both by standardized test instruments for anxiety and depression as well as by electromyography. It was not as effective with severe anxiety and depression. In a study with adolescents self-reporting physical or emotional abuse, *yoga-nidrā* was effective in improving the subjects' performance on a mental health test battery.

In a cohort of wrestlers, *yoga-nidrā* helped the subjects improve their reaction times while wrestling by improving their focus and concentration.

In terms of psychosomatic disorders, a group of subjects suffering from tension headaches were carefully evaluated medically and then separated into experimental groups that received biofeedback treatment with electromyography or *yoga-nidrā*. The *yoga-nidrā* group experienced about the same degree of relief as the biofeedback group.

A cohort of 75 female subjects with menstrual irregularities achieved a substantial rebalancing of reproductive hormones with *yoga-nidrā* compared to a similar sized control group. This result is consistent with the role of ordinary sleep in balancing many different hormonal systems.

Positron emission tomography (P.E.T. scan) studies by [18] demonstrated a 65% increase in endogenous dopamine levels in the ventral striatum of subjects Lou et al. [19].

One study of pain responses to colonoscopy carried out with music therapy and with *yoga-nidrā* compared a control group who received no intervention to groups who received music therapy and *yoga-nidrā*. They found that both pain and insertion difficulty were significantly less in the *yoga-nidrā* and the music therapy groups compared to controls. Use of *yoga-nidrā* with pain treatment appears to be an important future field of study.

An array of studies of cardiovascular and inflammatory conditions demonstrated the expected reductions in blood pressure and increases in heart rate variability, but also showed significant improvements in erythrocyte sedimentation rate, an indicator of acute inflammation, as well as increases in both hemoglobin and overall leukocyte count, both of which support better immune function. When *yoga-nidrā* was studied against other yoga practices (*prāṇāyāma, āsana,* meditation) it produced significantly better results.

A study of type II diabetics using *yoga-nidrā* in addition to oral hypoglycemic medications compared to a group using the medications alone showed considerable additional reductions in several blood sugar measurements. This is consistent with the well-known role of sleep in the regulation of blood sugar, appetite and satiety.

Several studies demonstrated significant improvements in most sleep parameters, including significant reductions in salivary cortisol levels, an indicator of stress. Datta et al. [20] reported such positive results that they concluded *yoga-nidrā* alone may be sufficient to cure chronic insomnia.

One contemporary form of *yoga-nidrā*, the iRest protocol developed by Richard Miller [15], has shown considerable promise as a therapy for post-traumatic stress disorder. It is the subject of major multicenter trial for use with military veterans by the Veterans Administration of the United States.

One effect cited by some yoga teachers is that one hour of *yoga-nidrā* is the equivalent of up to four hours of ordinary sleep. This kind of sleep dosage effect has never been established empirically, although anecdotal evidence suggests that the practice, done over long periods of time, does gradually reduce one's natural appetite for sleep (what sleep scientists refer to as "sleep debt," the tiredness we feel when our body is ready to sleep).

Given the example of Swāmī Veda Bhāratī, who appeared to have remained in *yoga-nidrā* most of the time in his later years, and who lived cheerfully and actively while experiencing very severe type I diabetes, severe cardiovascular disease and chronic pain, it would seem that *yoga-nidrā* holds much promise as an intervention in a broad range of health problems. Like clinical hypnosis, it is likely to prove useful with psycho-somatic conditions and auto-immune diseases, which are almost always associated with elevated levels of arousal and physiological stress.

7. Conclusion

Although it has existed as a practice in the caves of the Himalayas for centuries, *yoga-nidrā* has been widely available in the larger world for 54 years. It holds very significant potential benefits as a component in treatment utilizing yoga therapy for a broad range of conditions. In fact, this author would argue that it focuses and potentiates the already powerful healing properties of ordinary sleep. As both research investigation and clinical utilization of *yoga-nidrā* proceed, it's skillful use necessitates that we remember that *yoga-nidrā* is a state of mind which can be reached by any of the preparatory relaxation practices available today. Success in its performance requires repeated practice over an extended period of time in the context of a yogic life which gradually brings the practitioner to a continual state of profound and mindful relaxation and regeneration.

Acknowledgements

Acknowledgement is due to Swāmī Rāma of the Himālayas and Swāmī Veda Bhāratī (Uṣarbudh Ārya D.Litt.) for tangible and intangible guidance in yoga and specifically in *yoga-nidrā* over 52 years. Their interest not only in the practice but also in the rigorous scientific investigation of the practice and its benefits inspired this author to re-explore neuroscience after a career as a psychotherapist and professor. Their effort left us all an enduring gift of healing for humanity.

Conflicts of interest

There are no conflicts of interest.

Author details

Stephen Parker
Counseling and Psychological Services, Saint Mary's University of Minnesota Graduate Center, Minneapolis, MN, USA

*Address all correspondence to: parkpsych@yahoo.com

References

[1] Greene E, Greene A. Beyond Biofeedback. San Francisco, CA: Delacorte Press; 1977

[2] Rama S. Path of Fire and Light Volume II: Advanced Practices in Yoga. Honesdale, PA: Himalayan International Institute; 1988

[3] Bhāratī SV. Yogi in the Lab. Second ed. Rishikesh, India: Himalayan Publications Trust; 2019

[4] Bhāratī SV. My Experiments with *Yoga nidra*. Rishikesh, India: Himalayan Publications Trust; 2014

[5] Parker S, Bhāratī SV, Fernandez M. Defining *yoga-nidra*: Traditional accounts, physiological research, and future directions. International Journal of Yoga Therapy. 2013;*23*(1):11-16

[6] Arya U. The Yoga Sutras of Patañjali with the Exposition of Vyasa: A Translation and Commentary: Vol. I Samādhi-pāda. Honesdale, PA: Himalayan Insitute; 1986

[7] Parker S. Yoga-nidrā: An opportunity for collaboration to extend the science of sleep states. Sleep and Vigilance. 2018;**1**:57-63. DOI: 10.1007/s41782-017-0026-5

[8] Parker S. Training attention for conscious non-REM sleep: The yogic technique of yoga nidrā and its implications for neuroscience. Progress in Brain Research. 2019, 2019;**244**:255-272. DOI: 10.1016/bs.pbr.2018.10.016

[9] Pandi-Perumal SR, Spence DW, Srivastava N, Kanchibhotla D, Kumar K, Sharma GS, et al. The origin and clinical relevance of yoga nidra. Sleep and Vigilance. 2022;**6**(1):61-84. DOI: 10.1007/s41782-022-00202-7

[10] Sharpe E, Lacombe A, Butler M, Hanes D, Bradley R. A closer look at *yoga nidra*: A sleep lab protocol. International Journal of Yoga Therapy. 2021;**31**(1):XX-XX. DOI: 10.17761/2021-D-20-00004

[11] Bhāratī SV. The Yoga Sutras of Patañjali with the Exposition of Vyasa: A Translation and Commentary: Vol. II. Sādhana-pāda. Delhi, India: Motilal Banarsidass; 2001

[12] Lakshmanjoo S. Shiva Sutras: The Supreme Awakening, with the Commentary of Kṣemarāja. Culver City, CA: Universal Shaiva Fellowship; 2002

[13] Desai K. Yoga vidra: The Art of Transformational Sleep. Lake Geneva, WI: Lotus Press; 2017

[14] Niranjanananda S. *Yoga nidra*. Munger, India: Yoga Publications Trust; 1998. p. 2009

[15] Miller R. *Yoga nidra*: The iRest Meditative Practice for Deep Relaxation and Healing. Louisville, CO: Sounds True Publications; 2022

[16] Parker S. Clearing the Path, the Yoga Way to a Clear and Pleasant Mind: Patañjali, Neuroscience and Emotion. Minneapolis, MN: AHYMSA Publishers; 2017

[17] Breus M. How sleep impacts your mental and physical well-being. 2013. Available from: www.thesleepdoctor.com

[18] Kjaer TW, Bertelsen C, Piccini P, Brooks D, Alving J, Lou HC. Increased dopamine tone during meditation-induced change of consciousness. Brain research Cognitive Brain Research. 2002;**13**(2):255-259. DOI: 10.1016/s0926-6410(01)00106-9

[19] Lou HC, Kjaer TW, Friberg L, Wildschiodtz G, Holm S, Nowak M. A 15O-H2O PET study of meditation and the resting state of normal consciousness. Human Brain Mapping. 1999;7(2):98-105. DOI: 10.1002/(SICI)1097-0193(1999)7:2<98::AID-HBM3>3.0.CO;2-M

[20] Datta K, Tripathi M, Verma M, Masiwal D, Mallick HN. Yoga nidra practice shows improvement in sleep in patients with chronic insomnia: A randomized controlled trial. National Medical Journal of India. 2021;**34**(3): 143-150. DOI: 10.25259/NMJI_63_19

Chapter 5

Yoga, Mind-Body Coherence, and Zen

Junling Gao and Hin Hung Sik

Abstract

Eastern meditative traditions, such as yoga, Qigong, Tibetan Buddhism, and Zen/Chan, have long underscored the interplay of mind and body, and this mind-body problem is gaining empirical support through modern neuroscience. Our recent studies reveal a tangible link between the brain's electrical activity and the heart's rhythm, exemplifying the mind-body synergy. This chapter covers topics that Yoga integrates breath and posture to unify mind, body, and the environment; and furthermore, Zen/Chan meditation directly aims to dismantle all conceptual illusions, including those of self and universe, sharpening the practitioner's mental acuity, and challenging their perception of reality. This chapter explores the mind-body nexus and contrasts various meditative disciplines, primarily focusing on the nuances between Yoga and Zen/Chan meditation.

Keywords: yoga, mind-body coherence, Zen/Chan, brain-heart connectivity, EEG

1. Introduction

1.1 The concept of mind-body unity in Yoga philosophy

Yoga originated in ancient India, and it is grounded in the Yoga Sutras of Patanjali [1]. This holistic philosophy posits the unity of the body, mind, and spirit in humans. The practice of Yoga can lead to spiritual liberation or enlightenment, which is a pure state of consciousness and an Elysian spiritual state. A unity of the mind and body is emphasized in Yoga philosophy, extending to unity with other beings and our surroundings, and ultimately, a reunion of the self with the universe. The Yoga concept of Advaita, akin to nondualism, states that the true nature of the self mirrors the essence of the universe. However, due to avidya or ignorance, secular individuals harbor an illusion of separation between the self and others [2].

The dispelling of this illusion or avidya can be achieved only through the practice of Yoga, which includes physical postures (asanas), breathing exercises (pranayama), meditation, and other spiritual practices [3, 4]. Why is spiritual liberation pursued through physical and breathing training, rather than philosophical thinking and logical deduction? This stems from the ancient law of cause and effect, which asserts that all substantive actions entail consequences [5], and physical action can have a more practical effect than pure philosophical thinking. Moreover, the physical state of the body is intertwined with, if not determinative of, the mental state [6, 7]. Therefore, the practice of Yoga seeks to purify the body and mind simultaneously, foster positive causal effects, and facilitate the attainment of greater physical happiness and spiritual growth.

Once the physical aspect of the body is well-trained and largely purified, the focus of practice moves on to spiritual exercises and purification. The philosophy of Yoga places particular emphasis on moral behavior and character, referred to as yamas and niyamas. Yamas incorporate principles such as non-violence, sincerity, and non-theft, while niyamas include principles such as cleanliness, contentment, and self-discipline [8]. Adhering to these moral standards is an inevitable manifestation of their practical implementation in real life. If practitioners genuinely embrace Advaita's "non-two" or "nondualism," they recognize that the self and the universe are not independent entities but interdependent and unified. There is no need for deception or theft as these acts are inappropriate and unnecessary [9].

Following the rule of causality, only the practice of Yoga with substantial action, including both the physical and mental training, can help us purify them as a unity. Training of either the body or the mind alone cannot overcome the illusion of dualistic separation. The combined physical and mental practice of Yoga helps the practitioner cultivate a sense of unity with all existence. Eventually, consciousness of the true nature of the self and the universe will appear and merge as the ultimate reality. This non-dualistic philosophy is closely related to the concept of Brahman as the source of existence and the cosmos. It is assumed that the true nature of the self is identical to the nature of Brahman. The ultimate goal of human existence is to realize this universal truth and achieve liberation and enlightenment [10].

Over thousands of years of development, yoga training has formed an integrated system that includes body posture (asanas), breath control (pranayama), sensory withdrawal (pratyahara), focused attention(dharana), deep meditation (dhyana), the highest state of absorption or superconsciousness (samadhi). There is ethical guidance all through the Yoga practices. Yoga's body movements are designed to balance different aspects of the practitioner's physiology, promote physical health and vitality, and prepare for meditation. Breathing training plays a particularly important role in the systematic training of yoga, where the practice of breathing in and out harmonizes the flow of life force (prana), calms the mind, and regulates emotional states [11]. Both yoga and the modern fashionable mindfulness place a special emphasis on breathing [12, 13]. From a neuroscientific point of view, breathing training lies in the effectiveness of any mental training, especially with its profound physiological basis (**Figure 1**).

Breath training, or "pranayama," as respiratory activity can act as a bridge, spanning the chasm between the conscious and unconscious realms, uniting them into a harmonious existence. The Sanskrit term "pranayama" combines "prana," representing life energy or breath and "ayama," denoting expansion or extension. Thus, pranayama encompasses the essence of breath control in yoga practice, serving as a critical element in yoga training. In yoga, conscious control of breathing can be considered a conduit, linking the conscious mind with physiological processes typically unconscious [14, 15]. This unique interaction can serve as a direct reminder of our innate ability to influence our physiological states through mindfulness observation. The continual inflow and outflow of breath provide a flexible and vivid phenomenon for observation, much like focused attention meditation, thereby helping to anchor our attention in the present moment and with our physical body [16, 17]. This focus on the breath can serve as a robust defense against the mental wandering or even storm in our brain that occasionally arises in our minds, granting us calmness. The relationship between physiological and psychological processes is characterized by distinct temporal dynamics. Cognitive

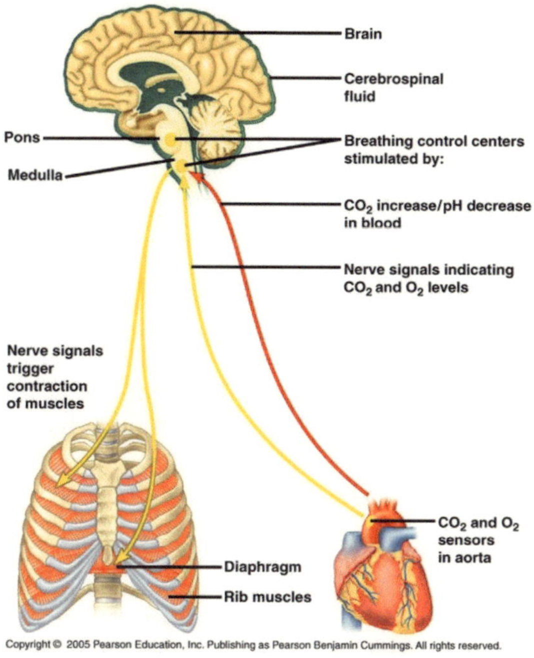

Figure 1.
The nervous control on respiratory activities.

functions generally operate at a more rapid pace compared to somatic responses, which are inherently slower and exhibit a finite range of adaptability. For instance, the human mind is capable of swiftly traversing a broad spectrum of thoughts and imaginings, often detaching from the present moment and engaging with abstract concepts or hypothetical scenarios. In contrast, the physical body is anchored here and now, constrained by the temporal and spatial limitations inherent to biological processes. By consciously coordinating breath and movement in yoga practice, we can gradually cultivate mind-body coherence. This resonance of physical and mental activities can guide the harmonious operation of our life energy, ultimately enabling our minds to become more focused, balanced, and harmonious [18].

Conscious breathing training can eventually make the mind to be more coherent with the natural rhythm of the biological body. It harmonizes psychological and physiological activities and achieves a state of effortless mastery. Once the mind can freely collide with and utilize this primal force, the union of mind and body can bring forth enduring spiritual power. When breath and consciousness are in tune, we become aware of the natural flow of our inner life force and experience how subjective consciousness can influence the physical state [19]. This "homecoming" simulates the process of our spirit returning to its roots, where the mind can release deeper insights and peace. Therefore, breath training can provide us with a journey back home—through the mind returning to the origin of the breath, ultimately retrieving our original intention [20]. This "homecoming" journey is realized through mindfulness-style breath training, bringing tranquility, unity, and joy [20]. By continuously practicing mindful breathing in yoga and cultivation, we can explore the operation of life energy within the body and establish harmonious interaction between physiological structure and subjective conscious experience. Pranayama provides us with a path to our inner rhythm [21].

Long-term practice of Pranayama and mindful breathing will increase the practitioner's interoception on the subtle interpenetration and merge between the physiological and psychological structures of human beings [22]. During the process, breathing is the bridge that can connect the conscious mind with the unconscious body. They have different rhythms by nature. Thus, breath can connect the primary physiological force of life and voluntary psychological control. With continuous practice, the boundary between the mind and body will gradually dissolve and be replaced by a macroscopic sense of unity. By deepening this cross-boundary link, we can touch upon the deeper layers of the self and experience the possibility of the self-transcending the mundane. The mind-body bridge established through the practice of mindful breathing is a solid starting point for exploring the inner realm and many other yogic practices. It closely joins the consciousness with the life force, endowing us with a transcendent form of existence [23]. Through it, we can strengthen the growth of the wisdom within the living body, and through this wisdom, return to the embrace of the supreme source of existence.

2. Brain-heart connection and neuroscience

Much of yoga's discourse has been fully described in other chapters of this book. This chapter will focus on the issue of mind-body unity based on the above discussion, especially from this novel perspective of modern neuroscience. The final part of the chapter will discuss other spiritual training, especially Zen Buddhism's, and their implication for yoga training and philosophical elicitation in terms of spirituality and enlightenment.

The interconnection between mind and body is a fundamental premise of various Eastern philosophies and practices, extending beyond yoga to include traditions such as Buddhism, qigong, tai chi, and traditional Chinese medicine. These systems all underline the inseparability of physical, mental, and spiritual wellness [24]. Till to date, these concepts largely resided within the realm of philosophical discourse and personal anecdote, lacking empirical validation. While practitioners and scholars spoke of the profound effects of these mind-body practices, objective evidence remain scarce. The emergence of modern neuroscience has started to shed light on the potential mechanisms underlying these age-old wisdom. With sophisticated tools to investigate brain processes and their relationships with bodily function, it is now possible to explore these concepts with scientific rigor [25].

Mind-body problem is the hard problem for philosophers and scientists. Nonetheless, the complexity of mind-body relationship can be partially elucidated through the relationship between the brain and the heart. Mind can be best researched upon the brain's responsibility. The heart, as a crucial organ, exemplifies the body's dynamic nature. Cardiac rhythm and strength continually adjust in response to bodily demands, and cessation of cardiac activity is the gold standard for the diagnosis of death in clinics. On the other hand, psychological measurement is complex, involving both subjective experiences and objective observations of brain activity. Although we cannot directly equate the electrical activity of the brain to mental processes, these electrical patterns are currently our closest approximation of mental activity [26–28]. For instance, stimulation of the brain's somatosensory and motor regions can elicit corresponding sensory and motor responses and subjective experience. Similarly, stimulating the temporal lobe can trigger patients to recall past events and even complex images. The seizures experienced by individuals with epilepsy provide compelling evidence for the relationship between brain electrical activity and psychological states [29]. Even though we cannot yet fully equate electrical brain activity with mental processes and acknowledging that various factors, such as neurotransmitters, continually influence brain activity, neuroimaging remains the most objective measure of mental activity so far [30, 31]. As neuroscience continues to advance, we expect that the accuracy and immediacy of these measurements will improve, opening up extensive opportunities for further exploration and measurement of mind and its interaction with the physical body.

Early stages of our neuroscience research discovered that heart-brain synchronicity is enhanced during mindfulness breathing exercises [32]. Mindfulness meditation, along with other Eastern traditions that include yoga, places emphasis on both mind-body training and the aspiration to achieve unity between mind and body. Two observable aspects of the mental training are trait and state, terms familiar within psychological theory. Trait refers to the long-term changes in one's temperament after practice, while state describes temporary changes occurring at the time of practice.

Our early studies found that mindfulness training can cause temporary state changes, including synergistic alterations in heart activity and brain activity during mindful breathing. These changes primarily reflect a harmonization of the activity and cardiac activity entropy in relevant areas. However, no difference was observed before and after an 8-week training period, indicating that while state-related physical and mental changes were identified, trait-related changes were not [32]. As analytical techniques continues to advance, subsequent research found that changes in alpha wave peaks and cardiac synergy metrics increased after 8 weeks of training. This implies that 8 weeks of mindfulness training can also yield long-term benefits on traits, dominated by a change in brain-heart interaction, measured by the correlation between the peak of the frontal alpha wave and heart coherence. Brain-heart connection may be more a sensitive index to monitor mental practice [13]. This suggests that short-term mindfulness breathing exercises can immediately alter the state of physical control in the human brain, while long-term mindfulness training effects changes in the frontal lobe, the control area of human brain cognition. This corroborates the age-old wisdom that immediate adjustments can alter the physical behavior of the body, but changing mental behavior requires a more prolonged experience (**Figure 2**).

Meanwhile, medical research and neuroscience also increasingly recognize the significance of mind-body integration, affirming the intricate interconnections between the brain and the heart. These interactions significantly influence cognitive function, emotions, and physiological processes [33, 34]. Also, our research probes into the potential links between our brain and heart, the fascinating dynamic rhythm they perform together in our physiology and psychology, and why the harmony between them matters so much to our health. Understanding these essential facts would spark fresh ideas on how one can bolster the coordination between the brain and heart through individual training, such as yoga and other meditation routines (**Figure 3**).

The brain and heart both have electrical activity. For example, brain has different electrical waveforms and exhibits different cognitive-emotional and arousal states. Mental concentration is accompanied by fast waves such as beta and gamma waves, and the relaxed awake state is accompanied to alpha waves. The heart generates its own electrical rhythm, which is further refined by signals from the autonomic nervous system. Therefore, two-way communication is achieved mainly through the autonomic nervous system (ANS) connection [35]. The vagus nerve is the main channel for information transmission, which transmits perceptual data about the state of the cardiovascular

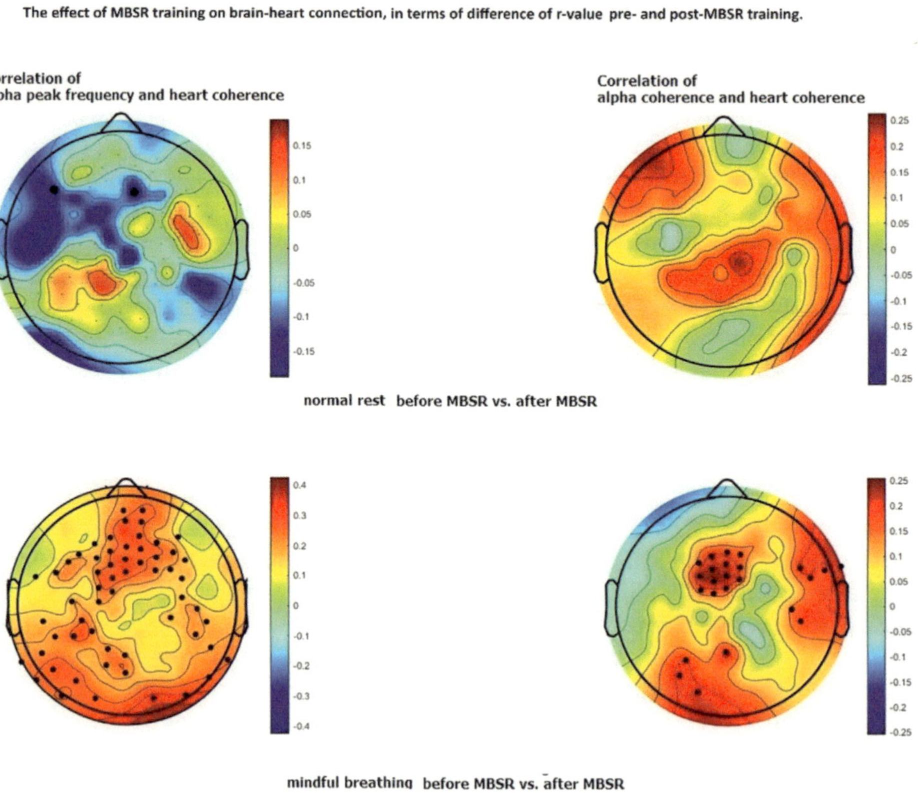

Figure 2.
Illustrates the brain-heart connections through maps. The connection strength (R-value) was determined by calculating the correlation between alpha peak frequency and heart coherence (left column), as well as the correlation between alpha coherence and heart coherence (right column). The upper row displays the normal rest control condition before and after an 8-week mindfulness-based stress reduction (MBSR) training, while the lower row represents the mindful breathing condition before and after MBSR training. The color indicates the differences in R-values before and after MBSR training. The black dots indicate electrodes with significant differences before and after MBSR training (p < 0.05, uncorrected) https://doi.org/10.3389/fnhum.2023.1008490.

system through neural pathways to brain regions such as the brainstem, amygdala, and insular cortex. Cortical structures, in turn, regulate heart rate and heart function through vagus output [36]. This rate and pattern of information transmission produces rhythmic oscillations that synchronize brain and heart activity, referred to as neuropsychological coordination phenomena.

In humans, the nervous system is divided into the central nervous system (CNS) and the peripheral nervous system (PNS). The CNS includes the human brain and spinal cord. The PNS is made up of the somatic nervous system, which controls voluntary skeletal muscles, and the autonomic nervous system, which controls the heart muscle, smooth muscle, and glands [37]. The autonomic nervous system is further divided into the sympathetic nervous system (SNS) for fight or flight responses and the parasympathetic nervous system (PNS) for rest and digestion. The main communication channel between the brain and the heart is *via* the vagus nerve, which belongs to the PNS. However, other neural pathways exist while play minor roles in brain-heart connection [38].

The heart itself contains complex networks of clusters of nerve cells (ganglionated plexi or GP) on the outer surfaces of the atria and ventricles. These networks, located

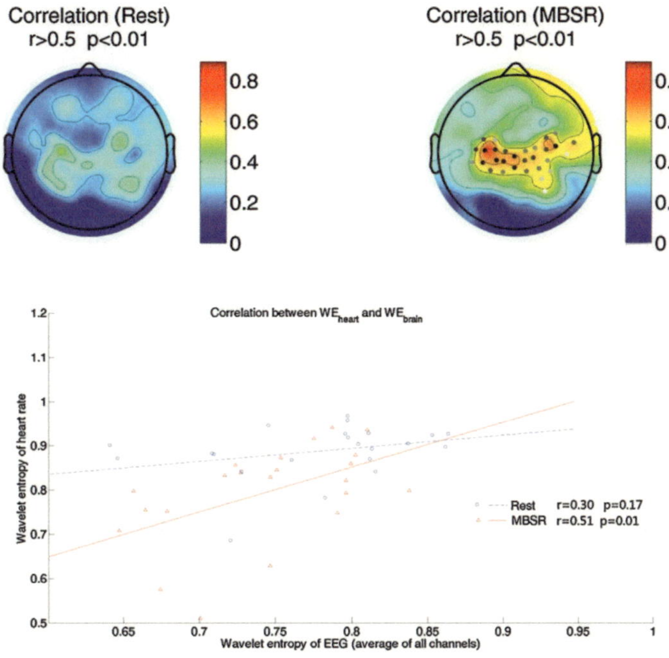

Figure 3.
Depicts the correlation between the entropy of whole brain EEG and the entropy of heart rate during MBSR practice (red line), contrasting with the absence of such correlation during normal rest (blue line). The small dots represent channels with significant correlation between HR entropy and each EEG channel. For a more detailed understanding of the color references in this figure legend, please refer to the web version of this article. https://doi.org/10.1016/j.neulet.2016.01.001.

within the epicardial fat pads, constitute the intrinsic cardiac autonomic nervous system. This system consists of interconnected GP, ganglia, and nerve fibers [39]. It interacts with the extrinsic cardiac autonomic nervous system, which originates from the brain. The intrinsic GP nerve networks likely function as integrative hubs that coordinate complex autonomic signals between the extrinsic and intrinsic cardiac nervous systems, allowing sophisticated control over cardiac functions [39].

These nerves establish extensive neural connections for bidirectional information transmission and feedback between the brain and heart. These anatomical structures serve as interfaces linking the central and autonomous nervous systems and participate in the sympathetic regulation of cardiovascular and abdominal organs. The sensory nerves of the cardiovascular system and the heart convey information about blood pressure, heart rate, respiration, and oxygenation to the brainstem area *via* the vagus nerve, including the subnuclear area. This area integrates these visceral sensory data and sends them to brain regions, such as the amygdala and the insular cortex. Conversely, the brain regulates heart function through the vagal motor pathway, originating in the medulla oblongata. The circular respiratory center including subnuclear area can further integrate the visceral sensory data and send them to other brain regions, such as the amygdala and the insular cortex [40]. The latter is related to emotion and can influence cognition eventually.

When EEG and ECG rhythms are synchronized and maintain a stable phase relationship, this is known as neurocardiac synchronization. It is characterized by the frequency of heart rate variability matching the EEG alpha waves. Neurocardiac synchronization forms the foundation of the brain-heart connection and significantly impacts physiological and psychological health [41]. The level of synchronization reflects the functional state of stress-related pathways. Different psychological states exhibit variations in synchronization with positive emotions and relaxed states showing higher harmony, while stress and anxiety are associated with dysregulation. As an indicator of overall resilience and adaptability, neurocardiac synchronization positively correlates with emotional stability and cognitive function [42].

Neuropsychological coordination aids in achieving emotional stability and the recovery from negative emotions. The extent of coordination can indicate how effectively the cerebral dopaminergic prefrontal lobe regulates the amygdala's emotional responses. Individuals with higher coordination levels experience lower anxiety and more robust positive emotions. Interestingly, in high-stress situations, such as combat training, individuals with greater neurocardiac coordination exhibit a reduced heart rate response and quicker recovery, indicating enhanced physiological resilience to stress [43]. A lack of brain-heart coordination often signals a poor clinical prognosis for conditions, such as depression.

Coordination between brain-heart rhythms positively correlates with emotional stability, cognitive enhancement, and increased physiological resilience. For instance, the balance between sympathetic and parasympathetic influences in heart rate variability affects emotional states with lower HRV in stress and depression [44]. Brain-heart connectivity significantly influences health, with ongoing studies revealing its impact on cognition, emotion, resilience, and clinical outcomes [45]. Higher cognitive readiness and capabilities are found to have a direct correlation with the index on synchronization of brain EEG alpha waves and heart rate variability with [46]. Enhanced brain-heart coordination is associated with improved performance in cognitive tasks, such as attention and memory, and this coordination is related to neurobiology of consciousness [47].

The disciplines of meditation and yoga always emphasize mind-body training that can confer benefits by optimizing neuropsychological coordination. This harmonization is considered one of the pivotal mechanisms contributing to their psychological and physiological advantages. Meditation, particularly the yoga practices is for cultivation of a synchronized relationship between the brain and the heart, which is believed to be crucial for deepening the mind-body connection. Generally, meditation practices are known to enhance the synergy between respiratory and circulatory rhythms, leading to a more coherent physiological state that supports overall well-being [48]. This improved synergy can result in a more efficient oxygen exchange and a calmer more rhythmic heartbeat, which together promote a state of relaxation and mental clarity [49]. Furthermore, the focused attention and mindfulness inherent in yoga and Zen meditation practices are instrumental in heightening inner awareness and interoception. This heightened awareness allows for a greater understanding of the body's internal signals, fostering a deeper connection with one's physiological states and emotional landscape [50]. Through these practices, individuals can develop a refined attunement to their internal experiences, contributing to improved self-regulation and presence.

3. Differences between Yoga and Zen meditation traditions

Although Zen and yoga both aim to foster mind-body integration and enlightenment, they adopt distinct methodologies and prioritize different aspects of the experience [50]. Nowadays, yoga often means training physical postures, but traditional yoga training involves much more on meditation and ethical living. The ultimate objective of yoga training is to merge individual consciousness with universal consciousness, and Yogis refers this as self-realization or enlightenment. Zen Buddhism, a unique branch of Mahayana Buddhism that appeared in China and later spread to Japan and other East Asian regions, diverges from this approach. Zen mainly focuses on practice known as "zazen" or seated meditation, and more uniquely Can-Hua-Tou, the inquiry meditation [51]. This form of meditation is central to Zen practice and is aimed at achieving deep states of absorption and insight.

The core practice of Zen Buddhism revolves around cultivating "mushin," a state of pure consciousness devoid of conceptual thought. Zen practitioners often employ short stories or paradoxical anecdotes known as koans to trigger this state and to illustrate the nonconceptual essence of reality [52]. Zen Buddhism prioritizes the attainment of direct experiential insight, downplaying the value of theoretical knowledge and eschewing superfluous and elaborate religious ceremonies. The ultimate aim of Zen is satori, a sudden flash of profound realization or awakening. This moment of enlightenment unveils the "true nature" of reality and the self, affirming that ordinary life itself embodies enlightenment. Zen and yoga, while distinct in their practices, both seek to engage practitioners into a direct yet profound experience of reality and self-awareness that transcends daily thought patterns. Both of the practices encourage and cultivate the virtues of mindfulness, discipline, and ethical living, both in pursuit of inner serenity and balance. Nevertheless, yoga offers a comprehensive approach that includes physical postures, breathwork, and meditation, whereas Zen mainly focuses on meditation and mindfulness all through the daily living. Despite their different paths, both aim to illuminate the mind and enrich the spirit [53, 54].

In addition, Zen meditation, in particular, offers a distinctive cognitive flexibility that yoga practice may not have, also there is intensive mental inquiry. Intuitive inquiry meditation is a specialized Zen technique that employs the cognitive function of doubt to actively and intuitively investigate the concept of self. Our neuroscience research examined the effects of long-term intuitive inquiry meditation of Zen practice on brain responses to self-pattern processing. This research offered intriguing insights into how Zen practice influences self-concept and concept of Buddha belief and doubt [51]. It is a meditative practice characterized by persistent questioning and doubt, fostering deep introspection [55]. This method prompts practitioners to challenge and eventually relinquish all fixed ideas, including those of the Buddha and the self. Research indicates that intuitive inquiry meditation can specifically alter the brain's reaction to self-related concepts. When presented with images of themselves and the Buddha, seasoned monks exhibited a diminished neural response to their own image during meditation, but not to the image of the Buddha. This implies that for these practitioners, the meditation's focus has shifted more toward an internal conceptualization of "self," demonstrating a more flexible approach to processing self-identity [51]. The study's outcomes suggest that intuitive inquiry meditation (Zen Buddhism) leads to a more adaptable and detached mindset when engaging with the concept of self.

Figure, Zen monks show a more flexible brain activity when comparing Zen and normal condition-Fig. 5ERSP data from channel Fz exhibit differences between the two conditions when viewing pictures of the self. Significant differences were found at approximately 200 ms among monks ($p < 0.05$, FDR corrected). No significant interaction was found using ANOVA (**Figure 4**).

This aligns with Zen Buddhism's teachings on the wisdom of nonattachment and the transient nature of existence. It reveals that through prolonged practice, Zen

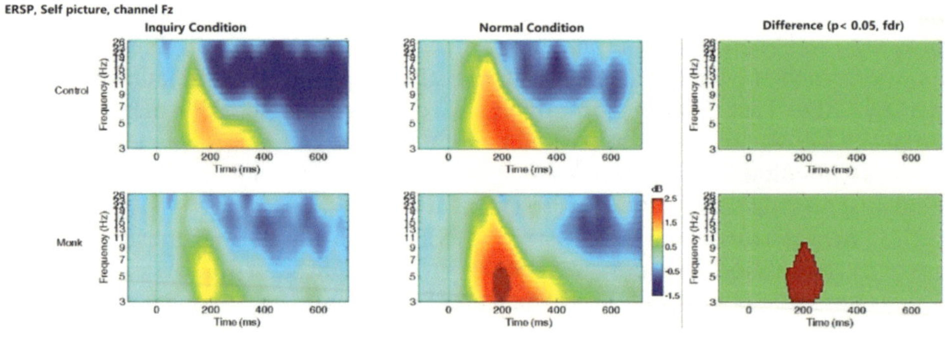

Figure 4.
ERSP data from channel Fz indicate differences between the two conditions when viewing self-pictures. Monks showed significant differences around 200 ms ($p < 0.05$, FDR corrected) https://doi.org/10.1016/j.heliyon.2023.e20075.

meditators can cultivate a mental state that enables them to swiftly move beyond self-identity, thereby attaining a profound comprehension of selflessness.

Zen Buddhism, thus, necessitates continuous meditation to train the mind for direct enlightenment (Satori) through immediate, intuitive understanding of reality's nature. It emphasizes the practice of meditation (zazen) and mindfulness in daily life to recognize the true essence of self and reality, transcending conceptual and dualistic thought. Enlightenment in Zen is often described as an awareness of one's own nature or Buddha nature, acknowledging the transience and interconnectivity of all existence, and understanding the fundamental emptiness of all phenomena [56].

4. Implications for health, wellbeing, and self-realization

This chapter offers valuable insights into the distinct approaches Zen and yoga take toward the concept of self and their potential effects on the brain's processing of self-patterns. It underscores the importance of further research in this field to enhance our comprehension of these ancient practices and their implications for mental health and well-being. The research also suggests that Zen Buddhism and yoga, while different, are complementary systems within Eastern philosophy, sharing similarities and possessing fundamental differences. Both of Yoga and Zen aim for the elevation of the human spirit and self-transcendence, yet they offer divergent interpretations of the ultimate goal and conceptual understanding. Yoga, stemming from the Sanskrit word "Yuj," meaning "to join" or "to unite," aspires to realize the union of the individual self (Atman) with the universal consciousness (Brahman). Through this union, practitioners aim to transcend egocentricity in the process of self-realization, acknowledging the interconnectedness of life and the unity between the individual and the cosmic self. This union is believed to bring about inner peace and equilibrium [57].

Conversely, Zen Buddhism's philosophy is nuanced differently. It underscores the concept of "emptiness" (Sunyata), a central tenet of Mahayana Buddhism and the essence of Zen. In this context, emptiness is not mere "nothingness" or "void," but a state denoting the absence of inherent or independent existence. It is an appreciation of phenomena that all elements, including the self and the universe, are interdependent and in constant change, devoid of any eternal, and unalterable essence [58].

From this vantage point, the primary distinction between Zen Buddhism and yoga lies in their perception of the end goal. Yoga seeks the "union" of dualities, whereas Zen Buddhism aims to transcend duality, directly experiencing the fundamental emptiness and interrelatedness of all things, leading to a profound realization of the impermanence and dynamic nature of reality. Zen Buddhism advocates for surpassing the final barrier to enter a state of "non-duality" or "absolute reality," transcending all concepts and illusions [58]. Within the theoretical framework of yoga, the individual self (Atman) and the cosmic self (Brahman) are viewed as distinct entities that can achieve "union." In contrast, Zen Buddhism emphasizes the inherent emptiness and interdependence of all phenomena, dismissing the notion of an independent, immutable "self" or "universe." In Zen, the non-dualistic awareness does not involve the fusion of two separate entities but rather a direct apprehension of the fundamental interconnectedness and mutual dependence of all existence.

While Zen Buddhism and yoga may seem to chart different paths, at their heart lies a shared quest for oneness, transcending the self-imposed boundaries of the individual ego. Yoga navigates through a dualistic lens seeking unity, whereas Zen Buddhism embraces a non-dualistic view that goes beyond such distinctions. This Zen perspective invites a profound shift in how we perceive our world, urging us to look past the mirage of separation and to appreciate the web of connections that bind everything together [59]. It is not just about grasping the fleeting nature of existence; it is about living in harmony with it finding tranquility in the very transience that defines life.

This essence of Zen is palpable in its practices, such as Zazen and Koan, where such non-dualistic truths are not just understood but lived moment to moment [60]. Meanwhile, emerging neurophilosophies have expanded our view beyond the brain-heart dialog to include a network of bodily communications, such as the gut-brain axis and the interplay between our breathing and heartbeat. Yet, even as science delves into the brain-heart connection with a reductive lens, it only scratches the surface of the profound interplay at work in the meditative traditions of Zen and yoga, where the dance of mind and body unfolds in layers far too intricate for simple models to capture.

In the practice of Zen Buddhism and yoga, this broader mind-body integration consciousness can only be implicitly recognized. For example, the practice of breath control in yoga, or pranayama, is seen not only as a way to regulate bodily processes but also as a way to achieve mental clarity and emotional calm. The practice of meditation sees a more holistic, systematic interweaving of physiological and cognitive processes, and more importantly, the interaction that collectively shapes our subjective experience. Zen Buddhism places particular emphasis on the direct role of mind consciousness and even enlightenment. Overall, both Zen Buddhism and yoga are effective tools for us to understand the world and the self and achieve self-transcendence. They offer two different but complementary perspectives that help us understand the nature of life and find peace and fulfillment (Ramsden). These philosophies may help modern people cope with the pressures of the multitude of tasks and the dizzying amount of information; after all, there is nothing new information in the world, mediocrity is self-inflicted, and all things are connected according to the philosophy of Yoga and Zen; There is no need of re-connection.

They provide complementary perspectives that help us grasp life's nature and find peace and fulfillment. In a world, where the pressures of numerous tasks and overwhelming information weigh heavily, these ancient practices offer us tremendous mental benefit and health.

Author details

Junling Gao* and Hin Hung Sik
Buddhist Practices and Counselling Science Lab, Centre of Buddhist Studies, The University of Hong Kong, Hong Kong

*Address all correspondence to: galeng@hku.hk

References

[1] Bryant EF, Patañjali. The Yoga sūtras of Patañjali: A New Edition, Translation, and Commentary with Insights from the Traditional Commentators. 1st ed. New York: North Point Press; 2009

[2] Raina S. The 'self' and the 'other' in Advaita Vedānta: Moral interpretation. Obnovljeni život. 2018;**73**(4):517-535. DOI: 10.31337/oz.73.4.6

[3] Desai MR, Patañjali. The Yoga-sūtras of Patanjali: A Commentary. 1st ed. Kolhapur: Prin. Desai Publication Trust; 1972

[4] Patañjali B, A., & Patañjali. The Light of the Soul: Its Science and Effect: A Paraphrase of the Yoga Sutras of Patañjali. New York London: Lucis Press; 1988

[5] Ramsden SCR. A brief overview comparing the core theories, cultivation practices and the interrelationships of Buddhism, Daoism, Brahmanism and yoga. Asian Culture and History Archives. 2022;**14**(1):16-54

[6] Bussing A, Michalsen A, Khalsa SB, Telles S, Sherman KJ. Effects of yoga on mental and physical health: A short summary of reviews. Evidence-based Complementary and Alternative Medicine. 2012;**2012**:165410. DOI: 10.1155/2012/165410

[7] Riley KE, Park CL, Wilson A, Sabo A, Antoni MH, Braun TD, et al. Improving physical and mental health in frontline mental health care providers: Yoga-based stress management versus cognitive behavioral stress management. Journal of Workplace Behavioral Health. 2017;**32**(1):26-48. DOI: 10.1080/15555240.2016.1261254

[8] Nandram SS, Bindlish PK, Sukhada, Shrestha AK. Spirituality led ethical decision making with yogic yamas and niyamas. Journal of Management Spirituality & Religion. 2022;**19**(3):237-257

[9] Bussing A, Bretz SV, Beerenbrock Y. Ethical principles of yoga philosophy in Western yoga practitioners: Validation of the Yama/Niyama questionnaire. Complementary Medicine Research. 2021;**28**(4):325-335. DOI: 10.1159/000513026

[10] Iyengar BKS, Evans JJ, Abrams DC. Light on Life: The Yoga Journey to Wholeness, Inner Peace, and Ultimate Freedom. Emmaus, Pa: Rodale; 2005

[11] Schmalzl L, Powers C, Zanesco AP, Yetz N, Groessl EJ, Saron CD. The effect of movement-focused and breath-focused yoga practice on stress parameters and sustained attention: A randomized controlled pilot study. Consciousness and Cognition. 2018;**65**:109-125. DOI: 10.1016/j.concog.2018.07.012

[12] Bloise PV, Andrade MC, Machado H, Andreoli SB. Increasing awareness and acceptance through mindfulness and somatic education movements. Advances in Mind-Body Medicine. 2016;**30**(4):4-7. Available from: https://www.ncbi.nlm.nih.gov/pubmed/27925606

[13] Gao J, Sun R, Leung HK, Roberts A, Wu BWY, Tsang EW, et al. Increased neurocardiological interplay after mindfulness meditation: A brain oscillation-based approach. Frontiers in Human Neuroscience. 2023;**17**:1008490. DOI: 10.3389/fnhum.2023.1008490

[14] He Y, Zhao C, Liu Y. Effects of respiratory muscle training on cough

function in neurological disorders: A systematic review with meta-analysis. Neuro Rehabilitation. 2021;**48**(4):441-449. DOI: 10.3233/NRE-210017

[15] Khoo MC. Modeling of autonomic control in sleep-disordered breathing. Cardiovascular Engineering. 2008;**8**(1):30-41. DOI: 10.1007/s10558-007-9041-9

[16] Ganesan S, Beyer E, Moffat B, Van Dam NT, Lorenzetti V, Zalesky A. Focused attention meditation in healthy adults: A systematic review and meta-analysis of cross-sectional functional MRI studies. Neuroscience and Biobehavioral Reviews. 2022;**141**:104846. DOI: 10.1016/j.neubiorev.2022.104846

[17] Lippelt DP, Hommel B, Colzato LS. Focused attention, open monitoring and loving kindness meditation: Effects on attention, conflict monitoring, and creativity—A review. Frontiers in Psychology. 2014;**5**:1083. DOI: 10.3389/fpsyg.2014.01083

[18] Feuerstein G. The Yoga Tradition: Its History, Literature, Philosophy, and Practice. 3rd ed. Chino Valley, Arizona: Hohm Press; 2008

[19] Chamberlin DE. The active inference model of coherence therapy. Frontiers in Human Neuroscience. 2022;**16**:955558. DOI: 10.3389/fnhum.2022.955558

[20] Nhat HN. The Miracle of Mindfulness: An Introduction to the Practice of Meditation. Boston: Beacon Press; 2016

[21] Stone M. The Inner Tradition of Yoga: A Guide to Yoga Philosophy for the Contemporary Practitioner Revised Edition. Boulder: Shambhala; 2018

[22] Gard T, Noggle JJ, Park CL, Vago DR, Wilson A. Potential self-regulatory mechanisms of yoga for psychological health. Frontiers in Human Neuroscience. 2014;**8**:770. DOI: ARTN 77010.3389/fnhum.2014.00770

[23] Jerath R, Barnes VA, Crawford MW. Mind-body response and neurophysiological changes during stress and meditation: Central role of homeostasis. Journal of Biological Regulators and Homeostatic Agents. 2014;**28**(4):545-554. Available from://WOS:000349064100001

[24] Payne P, Crane-Godreau MA. Meditative movement for depression and anxiety. Frontiers in Psychiatry. 2013;**4**:71. DOI: 10.3389/fpsyt.2013.00071

[25] Streeter CC, Gerbarg PL, Saper RB, Ciraulo DA, Brown RP. Effects of yoga on the autonomic nervous system, gamma-aminobutyric-acid, and allostasis in epilepsy, depression, and post-traumatic stress disorder. Medical Hypotheses. 2012;**78**(5):571-579. DOI: 10.1016/j.mehy.2012.01.021

[26] Gok Metin Z, Ejem D, Dionne-Odom JN, Turkman Y, Salvador C, Pamboukian S, et al. Mind-body interventions for individuals with heart failure: A systematic review of randomized trials. Journal of Cardiac Failure. 2018;**24**(3):186-201. DOI: 10.1016/j.cardfail.2017.09.008

[27] Kandel ER. Principles of Neural Science. 5th ed. New York: McGraw-Hill; 2013

[28] Zammuto M, Ottaviani C, Laghi F, Lonigro A. The heart in the mind: A systematic review and meta-analysis of the association between theory of mind and cardiac vagal tone. Frontiers in Physiology. 2021;**12**:611609. DOI: 10.3389/fphys.2021.611609

[29] Fisher RS, van Emde Boas W, Blume W, Elger C,

Genton P, Lee P, et al. Epileptic seizures and epilepsy: Definitions proposed by the international league against epilepsy (ILAE) and the International Bureau for Epilepsy (IBE). Epilepsia. 2005;**46**(4):470-472. DOI: 10.1111/j.0013-9580.2005.66104.x

[30] Chou YH, Sundman M, Whitson HE, Gaur P, Chu ML, Weingarten CP, et al. Maintenance and representation of mind wandering during resting-state fMRI. Scientific Reports. 2017;**7**:40722. DOI: 10.1038/srep40722

[31] Perlovsky LI. Neural mechanisms of the mind, Aristotle, Zadeh, and fMRI. IEEE Transactions on Neural Networks. 2010;**21**(5):718-733. DOI: 10.1109/TNN.2010.2041250

[32] Gao J, Fan J, Wu BW, Zhang Z, Chang C, Hung YS, et al. Entrainment of chaotic activities in brain and heart during MBSR mindfulness training. Neuroscience Letters. 2016;**616**:218-223. DOI: 10.1016/j.neulet.2016.01.001

[33] Jaen I, Fuentes-Sanchez N, Escrig MA, Suso-Ribera C, Reyes Del Paso G, Pastor MC. Covariate effects of resting heart rate variability on affective ratings and startle reflex during cognitive reappraisal of negative emotions. Cognition and Emotion. 2021;**35**(5):1039-1048. DOI: 10.1080/02699931.2021.1906209

[34] Thayer JF, Lane RD. Claude Bernard and the heart-brain connection: Further elaboration of a model of neurovisceral integration. Neuroscience and Biobehavioral Reviews. 2009;**33**(2):81-88. DOI: 10.1016/j.neubiorev.2008.08.004

[35] Williams PA, Rahmouni K. Crosstalk in the central autonomic neurocircuitry underlying cardiovascular and metabolic control. Federation of American Societies for Experimental Biology. 2022;**36**(S1):1-11. DOI: 10.1096/fasebj.2022.36.S1.R2542

[36] Kobrzycka A, Napora P, Pearson BL, Pierzchala-Koziec K, Szewczyk R, Wieczorek M. Peripheral and central compensatory mechanisms for impaired vagus nerve function during peripheral immune activation. Journal of Neuroinflammation. 2019;**16**(1):150. DOI: 10.1186/s12974-019-1544-y

[37] Beauchaine T. Vagal tone, development, and Gray's motivational theory: Toward an integrated model of autonomic nervous system functioning in psychopathology. Development and Psychopathology. 2001;**13**(2):183-214. DOI: 10.1017/s0954579401002012

[38] Waxman SG. Clinical Neuroanatomy. 29th ed. New York: McGraw-Hill; 2020

[39] Shen MJ, Zipes DP. Role of the autonomic nervous system in modulating cardiac arrhythmias. Circulation Research. 2014;**114**(6):1004-1021. DOI: 10.1161/CIRCRESAHA.113.302549

[40] Craig AD. How do you feel--now? The anterior insula and human awareness. Nature Reviews. Neuroscience. 2009;**10**(1):59-70. DOI: 10.1038/nrn2555

[41] Mishra V, Gautier NM, Glasscock E. Simultaneous video-EEG-ECG monitoring to identify neurocardiac dysfunction in mouse models of epilepsy. Journal of Visualized Experiments. 2018;**131**:57300. DOI: 10.3791/57300

[42] Mollakazemi MJ, Biswal D, Sunderam S, Patwardhan A. EEG segments synchronized to be temporally farthest from the R-waves in ECG are more informative during listening to music. Biomedical Signal Processing and Control. 2021;**68**:102660. DOI: 10.1016/j.bspc.2021.102660

[43] Dakal NA. Pedagogical technologies for the development of emotional and volitional stability in swimming lessons. Scientific Journal of National Pedagogical Dragomanov University. 2023;**1**(15):15-18

[44] McCraty R, Atkinson M, Tomasino D, Bradley RT. The coherent heart: Heart-brain interactions, psychophysiological coherence, and the emergence of system-wide order. Integral Review. 2009;**5**(2):10-115. Available from: https://www.heartmath.org/assets/uploads/2015/01/coherent-heart.pdf

[45] Deater-Deckard K, Bell MA. Maternal executive function, heart rate, and EEG alpha reactivity interact in the prediction of harsh parenting. Journal of Family Psychology. 2017;**31**(1):41-50. DOI: 10.1037/fam0000286

[46] Attar ET, Balasubramanian V, Subasi E, Kaya M. Stress analysis based on simultaneous heart rate variability and EEG monitoring. IEEE Journal of Translational Engineering in Health and Medicine. 2021;**9**:2700607. DOI: 10.1109/JTEHM.2021.3106803

[47] Candia-Rivera D. Brain-heart interactions in the neurobiology of consciousness. Current Research in Neurobiology. 2022;**3**:100050. DOI: 10.1016/j.crneur.2022.100050

[48] Sathyanarayanan G, Vengadavaradan A, Bharadwaj B. Role of yoga and mindfulness in severe mental illnesses: A narrative review. International Journal of Yoga. 2019;**12**(1):3-28

[49] Fiorentini A, Ora J, Tubani L. Autonomic system modification in Zen practitioners. Indian Journal of Medical Sciences. 2013;**67**(7-8):161-167. Available from: https://www.ncbi.nlm.nih.gov/pubmed/24469560

[50] Matko K, Sedlmeier P, Bringmann HC. Embodied cognition in meditation, yoga, and ethics-an experimental single-case study on the differential effects of four mind-body treatments. International Journal of Environmental Research and Public Health. 2022;**19**(18):11734. DOI: 10.3390/ijerph191811734

[51] Gao J, Leung HK, Wu BWY, Hung J, Chang C, Sik HH. Long-term practice of intuitive inquiry meditation modulates EEG dynamics during self-schema processing. Heliyon. 2023a;**9**(9):e20075. DOI: 10.1016/j.heliyon.2023.e20075

[52] Honda T. Case report: Zen meditation-integrated CBT normalized the impaired brain function of a chronic low back pain patient—From the findings of brain blood flow SPECT imaging. F1000Research. 2022;**11**:1384

[53] Acabchuk RL, Brisson JM, Park CL, Babbott-Bryan N, Parmelee OA, Johnson BT. Therapeutic effects of meditation, yoga, and mindfulness-based interventions for chronic symptoms of mild traumatic brain injury: A systematic review and meta-analysis. Applied Psychology. Health and Well-Being. 2021;**13**(1):34-62. DOI: 10.1111/aphw.12244

[54] Stritter W, Everding J, Luchte J, Eggert A, Seifert G. Yoga, meditation and mindfulness in pediatric oncology - A review of literature. Complementary Therapies in Medicine. 2021;**63**:102791. DOI: 10.1016/j.ctim.2021.102791

[55] Buswell RE Jr. The 'sensation of doubt' in east Asian zen Buddhism and some parallels with pāli accounts of meditation practice. Contemporary Buddhism. 2018;**19**(1):69-82

[56] Ishii S, Masuda A, Sargent K. Zen and Zen Buddhism: An Overview.

In: Handbook of Zen, Mindfulness, and Behavioral Health. Cham, Switzerland: Springer International Publishing; 2017. pp. 17-27

[57] Penumaka MPP. Luther and Shankara: Two ways of salvation in the Indian context. Dialog. 2006;**45**:252-262

[58] Austin JH. Zen and the Brain: Toward an Understanding of Meditation and Consciousness. Cambridge, Mass: MIT Press; 1998

[59] Kocot M. "The only way out is in": Transcending modernity and embracing interconnectedness in Gary Snyder and Kenneth white. Text Matters. 2022;**12**:249-268

[60] Sella Y. Non-duality in Zen-Buddhism. In: From Dualism to Oneness in Psychoanalysis: A Zen Perspective on the Mind-Body Question. Milton Park, Abingdon, Oxon; New York: Routledge; 2018

Chapter 6

Yoga Rehabilitation Theory: An Exploration into the Power to Heal Trauma

Sarah Green

Abstract

History documents the health benefits of yoga for self-healing and self-realisation. Yet how does yoga benefit individuals who have endured significant physiological, psychological and mental trauma? It can be argued that trauma frequently requires a re-adjustment to one's identity and their meaning of life, often connected to a self-healing and self-realisation framework. Yet, what role can yoga play? Accordingly, this chapter sets out to raise consciousness about yoga therapy principles in order to highlight, promote and inform such benefits. This chapter will draw on empirical discussions surrounding medical and social models of disability, as a way to highlight an increase need for awareness and acceptance of physiological, psychological and mental traumas through yoga. In conjunction, significant theoretical models underpin this narrative as a means of informing this emerging topic, specifically, Social Identity Theory (SIT), Self-Determination Theory (SDT) and Post-Traumatic Growth (PTG). The in-depth findings herein suggest that the novel concept of Yoga Rehabilitation Theory (YRT) understands the restorative power of yoga through identity adaptation, self-determination and positive transformations relating to meaning in life. It is suggested that the power of yoga resonates beyond a mind-body connection, to a deepening sense of purpose and transcendence for those that need it most.

Keywords: trauma, mind, rehabilitation, union, disability

1. Introduction

As a means of interpretation to strengthen the discussion in this chapter, key theories will be considered when assessing trauma initially and the ways in which yoga may aid an individual's rehabilitation. Namely, Social Identity Theory (SIT), Self-Determination Theory (SDT) and Post-Traumatic Growth (PTG). This chapter suggests that by connecting mind, body and spirit through mindful movement, individuals can experience an acceptance and understanding of the change that has taken place externally, to their body, and internally, to their sense of purpose. This is extremely significant in a rehabilitation framework set in a social context, where the focus is to accept and adapt, rather than fix and cure. There are therefore wider social implications to yoga as rehabilitation that encompass union of community for all individuals, irrespective of their ability—mental and physical.

Underpinning this discussion, is the recognition that in many societies throughout the globe, physiological, psychological and mental trauma are feared due to the wealth of stigma surrounding disability, as well as 'poor' mental and emotional health [1]. It can be suggested that such stigma may be increased by the medical model of disability. Such a model of disability is largely incorporated into the medical profession who work predominantly from a biological perspective. This means that, in this professional domain, disability is believed to be a biological outcome. Hence, there is mindset that the problems encountered by individuals with disabilities are relating to their physicality, in addition to individuals who have mental impairments. As a result, a vast majority of the medical profession do not consider the broader environments for such individuals. For example, the social, cultural, environmental and political landscapes that may challenge them ([2], p. 430). It is also claimed that the medical profession present an influential opinion in relation to the ideals of the human body, what it ought to look like and how it should perform.

In this manner, Gronvik [3] concurs that throughout history, disability has largely been seated in the possession of the medical professionals. The focus has been to see disability as a negative perception relating to lack of bodily ability and functions, rather than seeing the individual living with such an impairment. This rhetoric has therefore induced an entire medical vocabulary that focus on a body that is 'normal' and fully functioning, rather than a body that is different and can still function in an adaptive way. This has therefore created a powerful supremacy relating to disabled individuals and the idea that they are less able members of our society.

This is relevant to this discussion as a strong medical model discourse may in fact impinge an individual's ability to achieve self-healing and self-realisation through yoga. This is because when reflecting on the medical model of disability and its quest for a 'normal' body, there is little space for individuals who do not meet this criteria. Such individuals may be considered so different that they may not have access to yoga. In this way, the influence of the medical model of disability can influence the wider population's view of disability. For this reason, campaigners and scholars in disability rights strive to challenge heavily medical models that solely seek to treat, repair and normalise individuals who are living with physical and/or mental impairments [2, 4–6]. Campaigners and scholars have confronted such negative viewpoints by promoting the social model of disability, stating that societal attitudes and the built environment, rather than biological impairments, disable.

When considering yoga as therapy, it is therefore important to assert that yoga should be made accessible to all individuals, disabled and non-disabled. It is therefore relevant in this discussion to see, in what ways, yoga may be able to challenge the medical model of disability, to highlight what individuals can achieve post-physiological, psychological and mental trauma—creating an acceptance of disability through yoga, which will be more in line with a social constructionist view; one of union, acceptance and healing.

It could be said that it is a 'fact of life' and somewhat natural process of life course and world order that physiological, psychological and mental traumas occur, for whatever reason. It is therefore even more relevant to challenge such stigmatisation and fear through yoga as therapy as a means of creating acceptance of a disabled body, showing the rest of society that individuals can still achieve and may not need to be 'cured' or 'fixed', rather just accepted. In this way, it may be that yoga can also heal society's negative perception of physiological, psychological and mental trauma by acting as a tool to highlight and promote a greater sense of community and unity.

DOI: http://dx.doi.org/10.5772/intechopen.1003601

After all, a main facet of yoga is union—whether that be to unite oneself, to others, or to the wider world. Thus, it is applicable to see yoga as a tool to unite disabled and non-disabled communities.

It is in this way that in-depth discussions will herein take place, set within a social constructionist framework, to highlight yoga as therapy for individuals who have endured trauma, as well as challenging the negative conceptions of the need to 'fix', 'cure' or 'overcome' trauma. Underpinning this chapter therefore is the realisation that the understanding of yoga as union can challenge the negative perception of trauma (grounded in the medical model of disability) as a 'tragic' circumstance, into a positive perception of trauma (grounded in the social model of disability) as a 'transformative' circumstance.

2. Theoretical framework

As a means of interpretation to add to this discussion, key theories ought to be considered when assessing the impact of trauma initially and the ways in which yoga may aid an individual's rehabilitation. Namely, Social Identity Theory (SIT), Self-Determination Theory (SDT) and Post-traumatic Growth (PTG). As a way to develop this analytical framework and show the connections between such theoretical underpinnings, it is important to first consider each theory in its entirety before a wider discussion can begin on the emerging importance of their interactions in a yoga rehabilitation theory framework.

2.1 Social Identity Theory (SIT)

As a concept, the understanding of 'identity' is unique to each individual ([7], p. 1). In line with this, the expression 'social identity' highlights the parts of an individual associated with their group membership in society. As a result, it is recognised in extant literature that people as a whole have plural identities that is transient in nature and dependent on the environment or situation at that present time [8]. When an individual experiences physiological, psychological and/or mental trauma, their sense of social identity is affected [9]. This is especially the case as an individual's self-concept comes from his or her membership of a social group, as well as the ways in which the individual values and places emotional importance on such membership which is drastically challenged through significant trauma. Trauma to any level, as is mentioned, therefore dramatically effects an individual's identity, yet it is significant to see how yoga aids such challenges as a means of recovery in a "yoga therapy" context.

The main purpose here should be to analyse identity adaptation through participation in yoga. In this instance, it may be the individual's response to "who am I" after a traumatic injury that is benefitted from a therapeutic yoga rehabilitation pathway as a means of gaining acceptance after a significant injury. It may be the ways in which yoga acts as a tool to encourage a strong sense of social identity in the context of answering the question "Who am I?" that proports a notion that yoga, post physiological, psychological and mental trauma, instils an identity adaptation process and acts as a medium to aid an individual's rehabilitation, as well as an acceptance of physical changes that may have arisen during such trauma. In this manner, Yoga, as a movement process, can promote mind-body awareness and connection, encouraging individuals to appreciate what they still can do by the means of self-realisation ([10], p. 3). One of the most incredible benefits of practicing yoga is to be able to tune into subtle sensations and become attentive, which is unique for each individual. It is apparent therefore that individuals who are, in some form of recovery, develop such skills to enable them to realise their potential physically, mentally and emotionally.

Should yoga instil identity adaptation, individuals may be able to develop a strong sense of identity and a firm response to "who am I′. This is a significant facet in a therapy framework and a crucial turning point for an individual. This is because when an individual feels a sense of belonging, this transcends into their everyday life and their place within society and the wider world. A strong sense of identity may be developed through yoga participation as an individual can identify as someone that participates in yoga with others. They may meet other people in a similar situation to themselves, which would depreciate a sense of loneliness and overwhelm of the trauma into one of love and unity. This may sound very simple, but the subtle sensations that this may create aids empowerment, development and confidence—all of which are tools that can benefit individuals outside of a yoga practice and provide them with such a strong sense of identity and a voice within society. This is even more powerful as the individual may not consciously realise the power of a yoga practice overtly, rather just a sense of benefit to their emotional, psychological and physical health. It can be said that a depended sense of identity can promote a holistic sense of wellbeing as an individual may feel 'whole', complete and at peace with themselves, their trauma and world order.

2.2 Self-Determination Theory (SDT)

Self-Determination Theory (SDT) seeks to explore and shine light on an individual's stimulus and enthusiasm for certain situations that arise, recognising their unique driving factors that may be contextually, socially and inter-personally influenced ([11], p. 79). A deeper understanding indicates the individual's autonomy of choice to inform their behaviour [12]. That is to say, the extent a person has freedom to be self-motivated, which, in turn, influences their behaviour. It can be highlighted that the concepts that give rise to the notion of self-determination are autonomy, competence and relatedness ([13]: p. 311). SDT is extremely applicable when considering yoga as a rehabilitation tool because it considers the multiple constructs that, in this case, can be part of motivational experience to participate in yoga. Individuals may feel a determination to normalise their trauma through mind-body awareness, helping them to realise their potential and what their life can now be like [14].

The best way to achieve mind-body awareness is by active doing. Yoga therefore ought to be considered one of the most important tools in this context as not only is it manageable, affordable (as it does not rely on expensive equipment), but natural, innate and inherent to an individual deepening their understanding of themselves. In a recovery setting this is dramatic, and individuals may show a strong sense of determination to participate, should the environment and yoga practice be accessible. Determination is a strong characteristic to develop and aid a recovery process, helping people feel in more control of their situation and a stronger sense of choice in how to better their future. People often feel a strong sense to be able to return to some form of their previous life, whether that be their hobbies or physical pursuits. By developing a strong mind and body in yoga, individuals will have a greater chance of prospering in their rehabilitation and learn a skill that they can take further into life as a tool for their future.

2.3 Post-Traumatic Growth (PTG)

Post-Traumatic Growth (PTG) initiates a reflection on the ways in which an individual may experience mental and emotional transformations that are deemed positive after having experienced a traumatic life event. This can often lead to the individual's unique resolve being challenged, which can influence people to think differently about their sense of belonging and purpose in society and the wider world [9]. In other words, an individual's life course has changed, and they may need to adapt their identity as a means to find a place within their society, post-trauma. PTG therefore can occur as a deeply meaningful experience due to an improvement in one's outlook on life [15]. It is appropriate to consider how yoga therefore may indeed aid this process, enabling individuals to undergo a transformational process, which is deeply meaningful and shines light on a longstanding history of the way in which suffering can yield positive change.

Yoga as a mind-body-breath-connection tool ought to be considered the best tool to achieve PTG as the growth within oneself by participating naturally aligns to this theoretical framework. In other words, yoga helps people grow—physically, mentally and emotionally. In a rehabilitation setting, growth is significant as a way to develop pathways for each individual and promote longitudinal goals. From a linear perspective, this creates a trajectory to development and goal attainment that heightens identity and belonging, as well as acceptance.

The three theoretical concepts, detailed above, underpin this discussion on yoga therapy principles. This chapter suggests that when these three theoretical constructs interact and combine through the experience of yoga, new theoretical understandings can be uncovered. This chapter indicates that individuals adapt their identity to incorporate their trauma, become self-determined to regain a sense of normality and experience positive adaptations and PTG. The above connections are all influenced by participation in and the experience of yoga. This is because, individuals may appreciate that yoga helps them to re-establish their meaning of life. Analytically speaking, this relates to the ways in which participation in yoga connects intrinsically motivated factors.

It is important to continue these suggestions and move on to deeper explore the notion that the experience of yoga, in a rehabilitation framework, may be able to help individuals re-establish their meaning of life. It is recognised that traumatic injury or disability affects an individual's meaning of life and sense of purpose ([16]: p. 84). In connection, existing research and findings indicate that participation in physical activity creates changes in mental and emotional wellness, as well as quality of life that leads to a sense of empowerment [17, 18]. In addition to this, previous research also identifies that, after a significant injury, a person's sense of meaning, purpose and spiritual beliefs may change [19–23]. These suggestions are relevant in this context and can be used to establish a discussion on the perceived relationship between the experience of yoga and meaning of life as a means of appreciating the way yoga may create positive psychological states and self-growth.

The importance of this suggestion is to bring together previous research on trauma and spirituality with the emerging field of spirituality and adaptive yoga—a field that is underdeveloped and under-explored. Set in this context, it is important to examine this concept through the social constructionist lens as a backdrop to analyse an individual's dramatic change in their loss of physical, mental or emotional ability and how this impacts their self-esteem, confidence and meaning of life. It is in this way, as a yoga therapy framework, that individuals may gain positive experiences that "touch them in deep, mysterious and difficult-to-explain ways" ([24], p. xi). This could be because the experience of yoga helps individuals find purpose and meaning in their life through goal striving and goal attainment, both of which are unique to each individual. In greater detail, goal striving, and goal attainment is essential in a rehabilitation setting, to aid individuals. A goal, no matter how small, is significant and it is essential that should individuals need assistance mentally, physically or emotionally, to identify and achieve their goals, that it is provided holistically. Such opportunities should not be taken away from individuals, especially in societies that are steeped heavily in the medical model, where opportunities are not provided.

No matter what the individual's level of trauma or impairment may be, each person may develop a quest to re-establish their meaning of life, their spirituality. It is an intrinsic and natural reaction to such a change in one's life. Due to this, there has been an increased interest in spirituality in twenty-first-century and it has been recognised as an important facet of healthcare [25]. It is important to however recognise the unique and exclusive nature of its experience, which can be herein argued to be heightened by a yoga practice as a universal aspect of a human's psychosocial life ([16], p. 84). This may also be because there has been a greater sense of self established ([22], p. 817; [23], p. 1283; [16]). The power of yoga must therefore be recognised as an important way to help people feel at ease and find an inner peace and acceptance of their new situation. It may be that bodily changes have occurred, which instil a dramatic sense of loss of a former self and a grief process. Yoga has to be recognised to be able to fill this void and promote a sense of healing to find a new meaning to life for each individual.

3. Yoga Rehabilitation Theory

In very simple terms, yoga unites mind, body and spirit. To this end, physiological, psychological and mental trauma directly impacts an individual's mind, body and spirit; as their sense of meaning and purpose in life may change [9]. Yoga rehabilitation theory therefore seeks to recognise and understand the restorative power of yoga through identity adaptation, self-determination and positive adaptations. This is because, as this chapter suggests, it identifies the social implications of trauma, why they might be feared and explores how people may use yoga to overcome them. By connecting mind, body and spirit through mindful movement, individuals can experience an acceptance and understanding of the change that has taken place externally, to their body, and internally, to their sense of purpose. This is extremely significant in a rehabilitation framework set in a social context, where the focus is to accept and adapt, rather than fix and cure. There are therefore wider social implications to yoga as rehabilitation that encompass union of community for all individuals, irrespective of their ability—mental and physical.

4. Yoga as a prescription

If we are going to truly see yoga as therapy, we must now ensure that it is accessible to all individuals, irrespective of mental and physical impairments. This model of inclusive and adaptive yoga ought to be commissioned throughout the globe to ensure true unity. It may therefore entail a shift in perception from teachers, guides and followers in order to promote "yoga for all". Teachers may need to challenge their mindset and no longer focus on alignment and correct posture, but the configuration of each individual, for which feeling, and movement, is the most important. There may therefore need to be a shift in perception in this manner, where a yoga pose is a transient journey to reach inner and outer development, rather than a postural gain.

Teachers and guides must also be open to adapting their approach and style of teaching, this must be carried out in an emotional and caring manner, where pre-existing experience of working with vulnerable individuals may be beneficial. In this manner, prospective courses should be offered worldwide in order for teachers to specialise and learn how to deliver effective and inclusive yoga. Lessons should be delivered in a clear and concise manner, where individuals are free to express themselves, should they wish. Each class should be tailored in a person-centred approach, where feelings matter most and movement flows to connect mind and body, aiding the individual to explore their inner and outer strengths as well as enabling them to achieve true self actualisation.

To continue in this manner, it is understood that an unmistakeable facet of yoga is the development of breath, body and mind. The challenge here, when considering yoga as therapy, is to be able to guide yoga for individuals who may have some form of physical, emotional and/or mental impairment—to help them achieve the development of breath, body and mind. The teacher has to therefore be aware of themselves throughout the delivery of the yoga class, adapting their style and drawing on teaching methods such as mirroring, visualisation, story-telling, repetition and prompting. Not only this, but the built environment ought to be considered. Are classes physically accessible for individuals who use a wheelchair, for instance? The built environment is essential for accessibility and inclusivity, where all impairments ought to be catered for. Within this wider discussion, it is the way in which society ought to be required to change their built environment in order to cater for *all* individuals, to make sure that people do not miss out on the benefits of yoga. It can be celebrated that chair yoga and some forms of adaptive yoga are in place, however, the wider global perspective needs to be championed as a necessity to mankind, rather than individuals sitting on the edge of society.

5. Conclusion

This chapter explores a range of topics from disability rights and activism, to social identity, determination and purpose, as well as many other theoretical constructs. The greatest message is that yoga can be seen as unity, to unite mind-body for individuals who have sustained physiological, psychological and mental trauma and to unite disabled and non-disabled members of society, challenging stigmatisation and negative misconceptions of tragedy into transformation.

When considering yoga as therapy, this discussion strongly asserts that it is important for yoga to be made accessible to all individuals, disabled and non-disabled. It is therefore relevant that this discussion has explored in what ways yoga may be able to challenge the medical model of disability, to highlight what individuals can achieve post-physiological, psychological and mental trauma—creating an acceptance of disability through yoga, which will be more in line with a social constructionist view; one of union, acceptance and healing. Should this be achieved, the power of yoga can be seen to transcend beyond the individual, a transcendence that can only be described to reach the cellular level of mankind.

Author details

Sarah Green
Worldwide Independent Consultant, United Kingdom

*Address all correspondence to: sarah.e.green@hotmail.com

References

[1] Donoghue C. Challenging the authority of the medical definition of disability: An analysis of the resistance to the social constructionist paradigm. Disability and Society. 2003;**18**(2):199-208

[2] Brittain I. Perspectives of disability and their impact upon involvement in sport for people with disabilities at all levels. Journal of Sport & Social Issues. 2004;**28**(4):429-452

[3] Gronvik L. The fuzzy buzz word: Conceptualisations of disability in disability research classics. Sociology of Health and Illness. 2007;**29**(5):750-766

[4] Barnes C. The social model of disability: A sociological phenomenon ignored by sociologists? In: Shakespeare T, editor. The Disability Reader: Social Science Perspectives. London: Continuum; 1998. pp. 65-78

[5] Brittain I. Perspectives of Elite Athletes with Disabilities: Problems and Possibilities [unpublished PhD thesis]. Brunel University; 2002

[6] Oliver M. The Politics of Disablement. London: Macmillan Press; 1990

[7] Deaux K. Social Identity [Online]. 2001. Available from: http://www.utexas.edu/courses/stross/ant393b_flies/ARTICLES/identity.pdf [Accessed: 14 June 2023]

[8] Tajfel H, Turner JC. The social identity theory of inter-group behavior In Psychology of Intergroup Relations. Worchel, S. Austin, L.W. Chicago: Nelson-Hall; 1986

[9] Green S. The role of spirituality through adaptive sport in the identity adaptation of wounded Service personnel. International Journal of Therapy and Rehabilitation. 2012;**19**(9):516-520

[10] Frawley D. Yoga & Ayurveda. Self-Healing and Self Realisation. USA: Lotus; 2009

[11] Hagger M, Chatzisarantis N. Self-determination theory and the psychology of exercise. International Review of Sport and Exercise Psychology. 2008;**1**(1):79-103

[12] Deci EL, Ryan RM. Intrinsic Motivation and Self-Determination in Human Behaviour. New York: Plenum Press; 1985

[13] Hawkins BL, Cory AL, Crowe BM. Effects of participation in a paralympic military sports camp on injured service members. Therapeutic Recreational Journal XLV. 2011;**4**:309-325

[14] Wilson PM, Mack DE, Grattan KP. Understanding motivation for exercise: A self-determination theory perspective. Canadian Psychology. 2008;**49**:250-256

[15] Tedeschi RG, Calhoun LG. Posttraumatic Growth: Conceptual Foundation and Empirical Evidence. Philadelphia: Lawrence Associates; 2004

[16] Collicutt McGrath J. Posttraumatic growth and spirituality after brain injury. Brain Impairment. 2011;**12**(2):82-92

[17] Goodwin DL, Thurmeier R, Gustafson P. Reactions to the metaphors of disability: The mediating effects of physical activity. Adapted Physical Activity Quarterly. 2004;**21**:379-398

[18] Tasiemski T, Kennedy B, Gardner BP, Blaiklry RA. Athletic identity and sports

participation in people with spinal cord injury. Adapted Physical Activity Quarterly. 2004;**21**:364-378

[19] Boswell BB, Knight S, Hamer M. Disability and spirituality: A reciprocal relationship with implications for the rehabilitation process. Journal of Rehabilitation. 2001;**67**(4):20-25

[20] Boswell BB, Glacoff M, Hamer M, McChesney J, Knight S. Dance of disability and spirituality. Journal of Rehabilitation. 2007;**73**(4):33-40

[21] Faull K, Hills MD. The role of the spiritual dimension of the self as the prime determinant of health. Disability and Rehabilitation. 2006;**28**(11):729-740

[22] McColl MA, Bickenbach J, Johnston J, Nishihama S, Schumaker M, Smith K, et al. Changes in spiritual beliefs after traumatic disability. Archives of Physical Medicine and Rehabilitation. 2000;**81**:817-823

[23] Schulz EK. The meaning of spirituality for individuals with disabilities. Disability and Rehabilitation. 2005;**27**(21):1283-1295

[24] Hoffman SJ. Foreword. In: Parry J, Robinson S, Watson NJ, Nesti M, editors. Sport and Spirituality: An Introduction. Oxon: Routledge; 2007. pp. xi-xii

[25] Speck P, Higginson I, Addington-Hall J. Spiritual needs in health care. British Medical Journal. 2004;**329**:123

Chapter 7

The Feelings of Knowing – Fundamental Interoceptive Patterns Mindfulness-Based Proprioception Intervention (FoK-FIP MBPI)

Holly Pollard-Wright

Abstract

This chapter introduces the feelings of knowing - fundamental interoceptive patterns mindfulness-based proprioception intervention (FoK-FIP MBPI). This intervention correlates with the ancient and beneficial yoga practice through proprioception - based interventions, balance exercise, and focused attention training. It is based on the feelings of knowing - fundamental interoceptive patterns (FoK-FIP) theory which is both a theory of the mind and a unification theory that connects consciousness to physics developed through the FoK-FIP system. Collectively, theory and system represent an approach that embraces the importance of the meaning of "life" combined with new physics introduced into the peer-reviewed literature. This approach aims to stimulate novel avenues for disease treatment and prevention using expanded definitions to facilitate new ways of thinking about consciousness and its phenomena, including interoception dysfunction and emotional dysregulation. The FoK-FIP MBPI is a contemporary approach to wellness derived from the theory with a foundation based on philosophical insights and peer-reviewed scientific literature. It is the treatment for the feelings of knowing - fundamental interoceptive patterns disorder (FoK-FIP D), the maladaptive schema of the theory connecting disease to the cognitive force. Cognitive force and observing ego are synonymous terms for integrated perception (individual and generalized).

Keywords: mind, electromagnetic radiation (EMR) consciousness, cognitive force, feelings of knowing—fundamental interoceptive patterns mindfulness-based proprioception intervention (FoK-FIP MBPI), feelings of knowing—fundamental interoceptive patterns disorder (FoK-FIP D), interoception of FoK-FIP, awareness charge, awareness current, extremely low-frequency (ELF) magnetic field, ELF fundamental interoceptive patterns (FIP), FoK-FIP interference, FoK-FIP feeling tones

IntechOpen

1. Introduction

The feelings of knowing—fundamental interoceptive patterns mindfulness-based proprioception intervention (FoK-FIP MBPI) is based on a theory that includes a framework within a framework approach. The theory is called the feelings of knowing - fundamental interoceptive patterns (FoK-FIP) theory [1–4] developed through the FoK-FIP system [5], with both cellular and cosmological frameworks. The cellular frameworks occur through cosmological frameworks allowing the connection between physics and consciousness to be envisioned in new ways, including expanded definitions. The term 'new physics' refers to the theory's transdisciplinary modeling where the physical and nonphysical always co-occur. For example, where there is charge (e.g., magnetic, awareness, or electric), a current (e.g., magnetic, awareness, or electric) follows. The cosmological frameworks refer to the astrophysics and theoretical physics constructs (e.g., string theory) that, without mathematical language, conceptually expand the theory. In contrast, the cellular frameworks are the constructs represented by living organism models with DNA open to experimental trials. In this way, the FoK-FIP theory represents an efficient framework for understanding consciousness and its phenomena. Further, this theory's approach does something that has not been done previously. It paves the way to address one of string theory's biggest problems: its need for more contact with experiments [6]. The cognitive force is integral to how the theory's approach does this, representing aspects of the theory's expanded definitions and new physics introduced into the literature. In the FoK-FIP theory, the universe has five fundamental forces: electromagnetic, strong, weak, gravitational, and cognitive force. The theory also includes feelings of knowing - fundamental interoceptive patterns disorder (FoK-FIP D). FoK-FIP D refers to the disease of the cognitive force with abnormal sensitivity to the interoception of FoK-FIP. Transdisciplinary modeling using the theory's maladaptive schema gives an expanded definition of FoK [7], which is awareness charge and a *hidden variable* that fills with new physics knowledge gaps about what underlies interoception dysfunction and emotional dysregulation correlated to a broad range of animal models (human and non-human). The disease FoK-FIP D has the potential to broadly reframe scientific discussions that include physics and its laws and how those laws evolve by connecting them to medicine diagnosis and treatment. In this process, the theory deepens the understanding of the informal dictum, Life = Matter + Information [8].

Separation anxiety is an anxiety-related disorder common in dogs and is observed in the owner's real or perceived absence. This condition has been the literature's most commonly discussed canine anxiety disorder. However, etiology, treatment, and prevention remain elusive [9]. The FoK-FIP theory correlates separation anxiety with a type of FoK-FIP D (i.e., type I; see below). Aspects of the theory are being tested through an ongoing Institutional Animal Care and Use Committee-approved pilot study using dogs with anxiety conditions (PLAVS IACUC Number: C001). This research includes a daily intervention consisting of the FoK-FIP MBPI administered to the canine participants by their owners. This home-based daily intervention is derived from the FoK-FIP theory's transdisciplinary modeling that expands the understanding of quantum mechanics by connecting it to well-established rehabilitative interventions. As such, the intervention used in the pilot study is based on understanding linking the cognitive force to disease and treatment. Additionally, the FoK-FIP MBPI includes a novel use of neuromuscular electrical stimulation (NMES). The application of NMES represents a new form of exposure-like therapy as part of the FoK-FIP MBPI used to treat FoK-FIP D type I. In this process, the modality is used to induce emotional dysregulation in animal models (e.g., human and non-human) more reactive to stressors which could be broadly described as trait anxiety. In the pilot study, the owners combine NMES-induced emotional triggering with positive reinforcement (e.g., verbal praise and/or treats) to focus their dog's attention. At the same time, they guide their dog through proprioception and balance exercises in which their dog wears the NMES unit's associated pads attached to the skin on the abdomen. The ongoing pilot study has shown some encouraging findings regarding the efficacy of the FoK-FIP MBPI in treating anxiety conditions in dogs. Although the details of this study are beyond this chapter's scope, it shows how aspects of the FoK-FIP theory can lead to testable hypotheses, specific analysis, and experimental design. Importantly, this study represents transdisciplinary modeling, allowing the informal dictum equation Life = Matter + Information to acquire real explanatory and predictive power shown by ongoing research. The pilot study includes observations combined with infrared thermal imaging (IRT) through the testing environment to create baseline and post-intervention thermograms. This information is then correlated with the owner's daily subjective assessment of the change in their dog's behavior. The information gleaned from this pilot study will be used to guide the larger approved study "Feelings of Knowing-Fundamental Interoceptive Patterns-Disorder (FoK-FIP-D) in the Canine Model" (PLAVS IACUC Number: C001) using 60 dogs with anxiety conditions.

2. The FoK-FIP system's core components with fundamental concepts

- **The mind** is the fundamental entity with non-manifest potential that existed before the Big Bang and still exists. Through the mind's potential, a universe is manifested. Everything is derived from the mind [10]. The mind, which itself is not change, is the cause for change to manifest. Change with and without a pattern exists. The mind with no beginning or ending co-exists with the construct of time cognitively broadcast into existence that begins and ends.

- **The universe** described in the literature consists of approximately 68% dark energy, 27% dark matter, and 5% normal matter [11]. These are *attributes of the mind*. The universe has *five fundamental forces* which occur through attributes of the mind interacting: electromagnetic, strong, weak, gravitational, and cognitive force. Attributes of the mind have *states*: dark energy has a pure awareness state; dark matter, referred to in theory as focal points of dark matter (FPDMs), has a pure mental state; normal matter (also referred to as matter, or ordinary matter) has a state of mental images, and the cognitive force has a state of "distress."

- **Change** occurs through the mind manifesting its infinite potential in which attributes of the mind emerge. It refers to the attribute itself (e.g., dark energy, FPDMs, normal matter, and cognitive force). Change can be patternless or patterned based on the variation associated with the state (e.g., pure awareness, pure mental, mental images, or "distress") of the attribute that cannot be or can be directly or indirectly empirically measured. For example, FPDMs, normal matter, and cognitive force refer to patterned change, whereas dark energy is a patternless change. Further, *symmetry* refers to what the attribute with the state produces that cannot be or can be directly or indirectly empirically measured. It is associated with both transformation and the universe's fundamental forces. *Transformation* refers to metamorphosis (using an expanded definition) occurring through the mind's attributes, either induced through interaction or occurring spontaneously. It always includes change and can lead to a dramatic symmetry in form or appearance.

- **Consciousness** is electromagnetic radiation (EMR). EMR consciousness refers to information that can be cognitively broadcast. The EMR consciousness wavefront consists of the electromagnetic field. It is where the broadcasting of signals cognitively (i.e., cognitive broadcasting) by the cognitive force occurs.

- **The cognitive force** is both a synthesizing attribute of the mind and a fundamental force of the universe. It emerges through cosmological frameworks and is the "self" that cognitively broadcasts "life." The cognitive force is the perceiver of reality. It broadcasts signals derived from the electromagnetic field cognitively based on its sensitivity to the interoception of FoK-FIP. In this process, it models the components of interoceptive cognition consciousness, which is how the cognitive force learns. Further, there is only one cognitive force in the universe. However, it seems different because of how the universe is structured. In sum, the cognitive force represents the same kind of "self" that can cognitively broadcast "life" (i.e., interoceptive cognition consciousness) differently based on its sensitivity. Importantly, the cognitive force is not visible but exists as an invisible force through invisible dark matter (FPDMs) that came from the transformation of invisible dark energy. FPDMs can be scientifically inferred through gravity associated with dark energy, whereas the cognitive force is inferred from the behavior of living organism models. This behavior includes normal and abnormal obsessions, vigilance versus hypervigilance (that, over time, can lead to neuroticism).

- **Wave-particle duality of cognitive broadcasting** is the fundamental property of matter is that at one moment it appears as a wave and at another it acts like a particle. This ultimately depends on the viewpoint of the perceiver. In the FoK-FIP theory, the cognitive force is the perceiver with a sensitivity to the interoception of FoK-FIP (e.g., FoK-FIP interference or FoK-FIP feeling tones) that allows it to react so it can cognitively broadcast signals in a process that creates a viewpoint. The reactions of the cognitive force to the interoception of FoK-FIP are how it makes decisions. Cognitive broadcasting is a process that occurs through the wavefront in which awareness (i.e., charge and current) *melds* with magnetic (i.e., charge and current) and *mimics* electric (i.e., charge and current). In this process, the cognitive force broadcasts signals cognitively generated through the cosmological framework.

3. The core components of information processing

- **Feelings of knowing (FoK)** is a nonphysical awareness charge that leads to a nonphysical awareness current that can mimic a physical electric current [12], representing new physics.

- **Fundamental interoceptive patterns (FIP)** is the nonphysical extremely low-frequency (ELF) magnetic field produced through nonphysical awareness current. FIP is critical to cognitive broadcasting, in which its role is to push the cognitive force against gravity so that it can bind to the electromagnetic field.

- **FoK-FIP interference** is when the nonphysical awareness charge FoK through the nonphysical awareness current and the nonphysical ELF magnetic field FIP interfere with each other.

- **FoK-FIP feeling tones (e.g., pleasant, unpleasant, or neutral)** refer to the immediate and spontaneous awareness of the cognitive force with varying degrees of sensitivity to the frequency and intensity of FIP-FIP interference that occurs spontaneously.

- **The interoception of FoK-FIP** is a term that refers to both FoK-FIP interference and FoK-FIP feeling tones that form the substrate for cognitive broadcasting.

- **Cognitive broadcasting** is the process where signals derived from the electromagnetic field of EMR consciousness are broadcast cognitively by the cognitive force that reacts (e.g., automatically, impulsively, or with forethought)

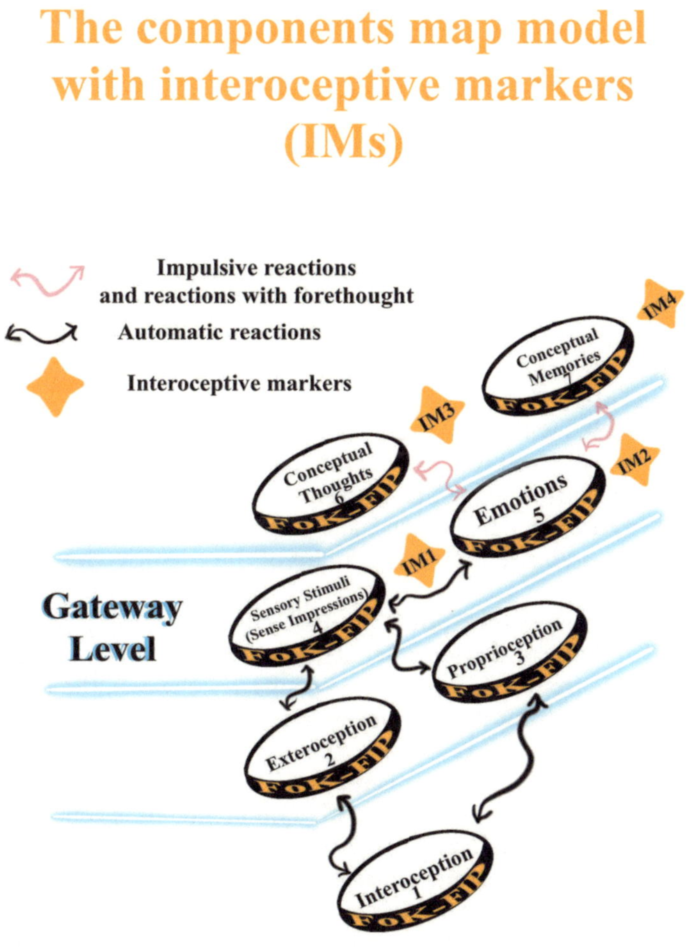

Figure 1.
The broadcasting of signals cognitively by the cognitive force produces components of interoceptive cognition consciousness (i.e., 1–7) envisioned through the components map model with IMs. The IMs show areas of susceptibility related to the cognitive force's awareness of its sensitivity to the interoception of FoK-FIP during cognitive broadcasting. The components map model with interoceptive markers (IMs).

to the interoception of FoK-FIP (e.g., FoK-FIP interference or FoK-FIP feeling tones). Responses of the cognitive force to FoK-FIP interference correlate with the consciousness percepts of attachment, aversion, or indifference (**Figure 1**).

- **Interoceptive cognition consciousness** is "life" and represents the smaller part of the larger EMR consciousness broadcast cognitively. This concept correlates to the famous series of lectures delivered in Dublin, Ireland, in 1943 by Erwin Schrödinger and in his influential book titled What is Life? [13]. Further, interoceptive cognition consciousness includes a phenomenal world cognitively broadcasted into existence by the cognitive force with myriad symmetries. As such, the history of the phenomenal world correlates with the stages of cognitive broadcasting occurring through the cognitive force that evolved to include higher-end cognition. The history of cognitive broadcasting is intimately connected to the "fossil radiation" called the Cosmic Microwave Background (CMB). Additionally, electromagnetic entities (i.e., living organism models with DNA) began emerging into the phenomenal world of interoceptive cognition consciousness when the cognitive force began broadcasting signals to create higher-end cognition.

- **Living organism models with DNA** are electromagnetic figures representing cellular frameworks that emerge within cosmological frameworks. Further, the sensitivity of the cognitive force of the framework to the interoception of FoK-FIP produces interoceptive cognition consciousness with a certain continuity. In this process, the distinctive way signals are cognitively broadcast by the cognitive force is represented by living organism models with DNA. Notably, when living organism models emerge into the phenomenal world, they are perceived by the cognitive force as if the world is projected around them. Additionally, the cognitive force cannot perceive itself directly. Instead, it is aware of FoK-FIP feeling tones and associates them with electromagnetic entities. In this process, the awareness of FoK-FIP feeling tones is how the cognitive force derives a "sense of self" that begins with an impression of cognitively broadcast senses that leads to higher-end cognitive broadcasting. Through FoK-FIP feeling tones, these electromagnetic entities have a distinctive élan that sets them apart as remarkable and special from the other "objects" and electromagnetic entities in the phenomenal world based on the viewpoint of the cognitive force.

- **EMR consciousness wavefront** is produced by the coupling between the nonphysical and physical electromagnetic field. The cognitive force is bound to parts of the wavefront. Further, in the cellular framework, the EMR consciousness wavefront exists based on the body of electromagnetic entities representing the framework. As such, the wavefront can be envisioned in myriad ways correlated with living organism models with DNA. For example, the EMR consciousness wavefront correlated with animal models is coupled to the central nervous system and peripheral nervous tissue in which the spinal cord connecting the body and brain is integral to the cognitive broadcasting process. The core concept here is that EMR consciousness is coupled to structures in which regions connect, allowing the wavefront to form so that cognitive broadcasting can occur.

- **The polarity of the cognitive force** is "bipolar," which does not match current definitions. Polarity represents new physics as the property of the cognitive force that emerges from FoK and is "pushed" by FIP. Cognitive broadcasting ultimately occurs through the cognitive force's polarity in which *intrinsic* polarity is derived from FoK whereas *extrinsic* polarity is derived from FIP.

- **Cognitive pixels** defined in the theory are "bits" of information in the EMR consciousness wavefront with cognitive force. The cognitive force with polarity (e.g., intrinsic and extrinsic) will cognitively bind to parts of the electromagnetic field while pushed by FIP in a process correlated with the binding process in the literature. Cognitive binding produces cognitive pixels that allow the cognitive force to act as a "cognitive magnet." Through the EMR consciousness wavefront, the cognitive force can "pull itself" together through billions of cognitive pixels brought together simultaneously. This process refers to the chunking and stimulus organization of cognitive pixels that generates the components of interoceptive cognition consciousness envisioned through the components map model with IMs.

- **The antecedent and the consequent**. The interoception of FoK-FIP is "the antecedent," and reactions to it are "the consequent" [14] related to cognitive broadcasting. The cognitive force's sensitivity to FoK-FIP feeling tones while broadcasting signals causes reactions that can lead to emotional processing. The cognitive broadcasting of signals produces "if-then" relationships that correlate to emotional biasing.

- **"Distress" = FoK + FIP,** in the theory. The "distress" of the cognitive force is one of the more significant domains of cognitive broadcasting, impacting a wide range of signal processing. It refers to the normal state of the cognitive force with varying normal and abnormal sensitivities to the interoception of FoK-FIP. In this modeling, "distress" is not always associated with dysfunction. Instead, through cognitive force, "distress" refers to the two-part relationship between "the consequent" (i.e., reacting) and "the antecedent" (i.e., FoK-FIP) that creates the "if-then" relationship of "fear" and "anxiety" required to make decisions. Further, the "Fear" of the cognitive force is an intervening variable between the FoK awareness charge and awareness current. Through FoK-FIP interference, awareness charge and current are the sets of context-dependent stimuli intensity and frequency [15]. They lead to the cognitive force's responses through automatic and impulsive reactions. In contrast, the "anxiety" of the cognitive force is the variable that follows FoK through FIP. It is intimately connected to feeling the patterns of the ELF field FIP associated with FoK-FIP feeling tones. Additionally, FIP is how impulse is experienced and integral to the memory of the cognitive force. Degrees of impulse that are experienced as if they were pushing causes the cognitive force to bind to parts of the electromagnetic field through cognitive binding. In sum, FoK refers to the "fear expression" of the cognitive force whereas "anxiety learning" occurs through ELF magnetic field FIP patterns. Higher-end cognitive broadcasting is how the "fear" and "anxiety" of the cognitive force manifests in complex ways related to living organisms with DNA, such as the behavioral responses of animal models with the "fight or flight" response.

- **A feedback loop of cognitive broadcasting** occurs through the reactions of the cognitive force to the interoception of FoK-FIP. It consists of an automatic reaction followed by an impulsive reaction representing a reaction sequence that "accelerates" cognitive broadcasting. Additionally, this response sequence drives "informativeness" [16], which might include broadcasting signals for emotional processing. Further, automatic reactions followed by impulsive reactions represent an over-practiced response that may or may not be followed by a reaction with forethought.

- **The "brake" and the "accelerator"**. The reaction with forethought represents the "brake" that inhibits the cognitive force's creation of "informativeness" through broadcasting for higher-end cognition. In this process, a reaction with forethought helps slow or stop the drive created through the automatic reaction that is followed by an impulsive reaction sequence. Importantly, higher-end cognitive broadcasting correlates the reactions of the cognitive force to the behavior of the electromagnetic entities that emerge in the phenomenal world of interoceptive cognition consciousness. For example, frameworks represented by electromagnetic entities of animal models have through their central nervous system an "accelerator" mechanism consisting of the major excitatory neurotransmitter glutamate and a "brake" mechanism through the major inhibitory neurotransmitters Gamma-aminobutyric acid (GABA) and glycine. In vertebrates, glutamate is the most abundant excitatory neurotransmitter and plays a critical role in memory, cognition, and mood regulation through its metabolism and several types of receptors throughout the central nervous system. In contrast, GABA and glycine are common inhibitory neurotransmitters associated with producing a calming effect by lessening the ability of a nerve cell to receive, create or send chemical messages to other nerve cells.

4. The cellular framework

The cellular frameworks of the FoK-FIP theory refer to the particular assembly of parts that facilitates cognitive broadcasting. At every moment in the cellular FoK-FIP frameworks, the stages of cognitive broadcasting occur through the activity of many trillions of cells with DNA. The FoK-gene expression causes the emergence of the cognitive force along with producing FIP. Further, cognitive broadcasting is not intrinsic to the particular assembly of the parts [17]. Instead, this process depends on the viewpoint of the cognitive force of the framework that defines signals cognitively by reacting to the interoception of FoK-FIP. The cognitive force's responses largely depend on its sensitivity to FoK-FIP interference without awareness or with awareness of FoK-FIP feeling tones. Importantly, the cells of a particular cellular framework can differ, but a core concept is that they all encode the same cognitive force through the expression of the FoK-gene. Additionally, cognitive broadcasting occurs through cycles correlated to cognitive cycles discussed in the literature [18]. In animal models, the parts of the cellular framework integral to cognitive broadcasting consist of a head, thorax, and abdominopelvic region connected through the EMR consciousness wavefront coupled to the spinal cord and peripheral nervous tissue. This connection includes the process where awareness current mimics the electric current of ions sodium, potassium, and chloride that muscles and nerves generate through contraction or signal transmission. In this process, the activity of "excitable tissues" [19] made of cells such as myocytes (e.g., smooth, cardiac, and skeletal) and neurons connect with the continuous production of the interoception of FoK-FIP. In the cellular framework, the interoception of FoK-FIP is produced continuously through the awareness charge FoK when the FoK-gene is expressed. This process leads to the continuous production of the ELF magnetic field FIP that melds with magnetic fields from other naturally occurring processes in the cellular framework.

The description of the components of the cellular framework that follows refers to human models, which correlates in many regards to dog models:

4.1 The thorax is the primary region for continuous FoK-FIP interference

In the cellular framework correlating with animal models, the thorax is considered the primary region in the body for the consistent production of FoK-FIP interference. In the human model, landmarks for this region include the suprasternal notch, which is the visible dip at the base of the neck between the two medial collarbones, the xiphoid process, which is roughly located in the ventral midline at the 9th–10th thoracic vertebra, and the nipple line. Magnetically sensitive organs, through the sensitive cognitive force pushed by the ELF magnetic field FIP, are located in the thoracic and abdominopelvic regions, congruent with cadaver research [20]. These organs include the heart [21], lung [22], spleen [23, 24], liver [25], and pancreas [26, 27]. Further, through the cellular framework, the death of cells occurs. *Apoptosis* is a normal and controlled aspect related to the functioning of the cellular framework. However, continuous cognitive broadcasting through the cognitive force is not interrupted even though cell death occurs. A core reason for this is the cardiovascular system, in which activation of the thoracic region correlates with the continuous generation of the interoception of FoK-FIP. The heart's myocytes play a significant role in this process. The specialized cardiac pacemaker cells control the heart's contraction. The heart is the organ in the thorax that correlates with consistent activation with aspects that cannot be controlled voluntarily. Involuntary movements associated with the thoracic region activation occur through cardiac muscle tissue. This activation includes specialized cardiac myocytes generating spontaneous action potentials correlated with FoK gene expression. Through this relationship, cardiac conduction corresponds with a rate of continuous production of the interoception of FoK-FIP through pacemaker cells located in the heart's sinoatrial (SA) and atrioventricular (AV) nodes. This concept includes FoK-FIP interference beginning in the thoracic region through the heart, which ultimately corresponds with unawareness of "distress." Through the cells located in the thoracic region, the cognitive force (i.e., individual and generalized integrated perception) continuously emerges simultaneously with the depolarization of cardiac cells or where synchronous firing occurs. Notably, in the thorax are the organs of circulation and respiration, in which the heart is the primary organ that is the "gatekeeper" of the process. The heart's continuous activity, including the activity of an artificial heart (e.g., artificial heart patients), ensures the connections needed to form the EMR consciousness wavefront allowing the cognitive force to broadcast signals cognitively.

The transdisciplinary modeling of the FoK-FIP theory builds on the discovery of a specific oxytocin (OT) system, including the presence of OT and the OT receptor (OTR) in rodents and human hearts [28]. OT exerts its functions by binding to OTRs in cardiac cells or indirectly in the vasculature to regulate function [29]. The left ventricular (LV) preload and the inotropic state [30] may decrease in this process. Further, OT induces vasoconstriction and vasodilation [31] depending on the vascular bed with which it interacts. Through the thoracic region in which cognitive broadcasting occurs, OT modulates social and emotional processes associated with many animal models [32]. In the FoK-FIP theory, integral to how OT modulation occurs is the EMR consciousness wavefront coupled to the central nervous system and peripheral nervous tissue. In this process, activation of the thoracic region includes continuous FoK-FIP interference production with OT control of vascular tone, blood flow, regrowth, and remodeling [33, 34]. Varying amounts of OT production in the brain/hypothalamus connects to the thorax region activation with the cognitive force through the EMR consciousness wavefront coupled to the central nervous system and peripheral nervous tissue. The broadcasting of signals cognitively by the cognitive force ultimately creates OT effects that correlate to "distress," in which the interoception of FoK-FIP acts as the antecedent, and the reactions are consequent. Through this relationship, the continuous production of "distress" signals (i.e., FoK-derived "fear" and FIP-derived "anxiety") has effects on the cognitive force related to cognitive broadcasting. Through higher-end cognitive broadcasting, the cognitive force that reacts correlates to the behavior of animal models. As such, the transdisciplinary modeling of the theory refers to new ways of understanding aspects of the behavior choices of animal models associated with goals and moral beliefs [35]. This behavior includes social stress and anxiety, social memory, affiliation and bonding, emotion recognition, mentalizing, empathy, and interpersonal trust [32].

4.2 The FoK-FIP signaling transduction pathway

The FoK-FIP signaling transduction pathway consists of an inner and outer layer and occurs through a general mass of cells. The *inner layer* correlated with human models consists of the brain and spinal cord coupled to the EMR consciousness wavefront and peripheral nervous tissue. The spinal cord is part of the inner transduction pathway that connects the head to the thorax and abdominopelvic regions. The connected components of the cellular framework allow the formation of the EMR consciousness wavefront. The brain represents the proximal part of the inner layer. Integral to this pathway is the brain stem [36], the thalamocortical system [37], and the frontal [38], striatal [39], and cerebellar regions [40, 41]. The signaling transduction pathway spreads through a zone of energetically charged particles from sensory cortices to rostral corticothalamic regions and the posterior frontal area [41]. In this process, the cortical and subcortical claustrum, including the anterior and posterior cortico-claustral tracts, connect the claustrum to the prefrontal cortex and visual areas [42]. The superior tract that links the claustrum with the sensorimotor cortex and the lateral pathway that connects the claustrum to the auditory cortex are included. A claustral medial pathway connects the claustrum with the basal ganglia [42]. Additionally, the inner layer of this pathway has a bilateral connection between the claustrum and contralateral cortical areas and interclaustral communication with interconnection bundles interspersed within the bulk of the trunk of the corpus callosum [42, 43]. In contrast, the *outer layer* of this pathway consists of the ganglia (e.g., superior cervical ganglion, first thoracic ganglion, celiac ganglion, superior mesenteric ganglion, first lumbar ganglion, inferior mesenteric ganglion, first sacral ganglion). It also includes the vagus and paired splenic nerves (e.g., cardiopulmonary, thoracic, lumbar, sacral, and pelvic splanchnic nerves).

4.3 The FoK-FIP signaling network

This network refers to connective tissue cells congruent with a schema to categorize tissue-specific types [20]. It includes fibrous connective tissue (e.g., skin, tendons, ligaments, aponeuroses), adipose connective tissue, and skeletal tissue (e.g., bone and cartilage). This signaling network can be further categorized according to the following criteria: The connective tissue is either layered between different types of tissue (e.g., epithelial, muscle, nerves) or surrounds tissues (e.g., blood vessels). It occupies the space between organs (e.g., subcutaneous, retroperitoneal). The

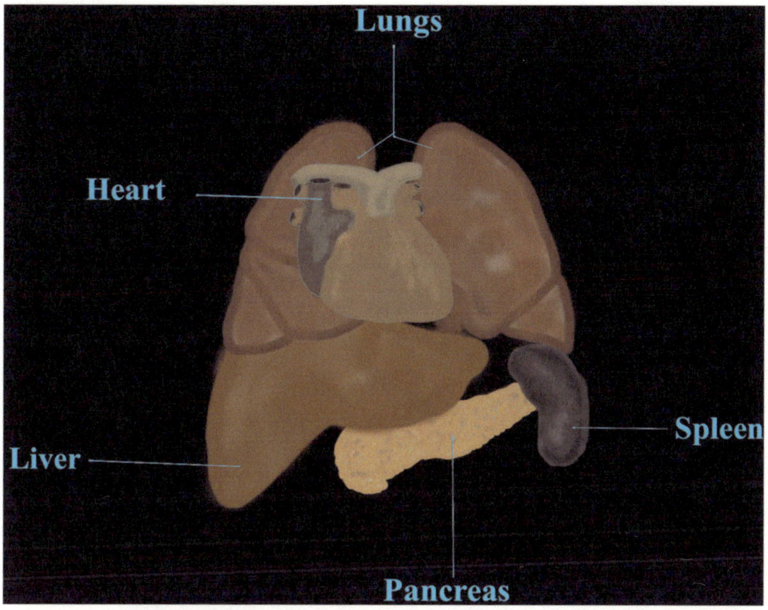

Figure 2.
The thoracic region includes the magnetically sensitive organs the heart, lung, spleen, liver, and pancreas through the cognitive force. The thoracic primary region in the human model.

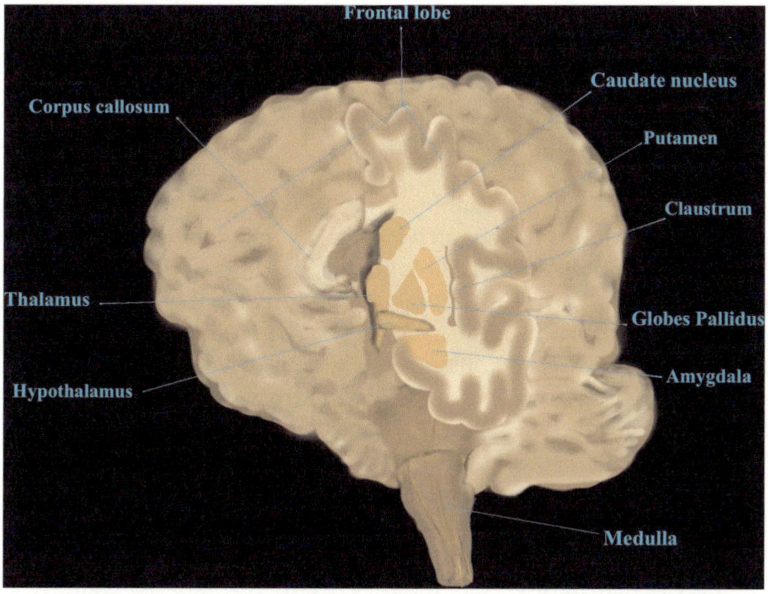

Figure 3.
The brain is part of the inner layer of the FoK-FIP signaling transduction pathway depicted here with the left hemisphere coronally sectioned at the level of the basal ganglia. These images were created by building upon the work of frank H. Netter, MD [48], and the John W. Sundsten institution, clay brain content: 2-D and 3-D views of the brain from cadaver sections, MRI scans, and computer reconstructions, *digital anatomist project (Seattle, WA: Department of Biological Structure, University of Washington, 1994). The brain.*

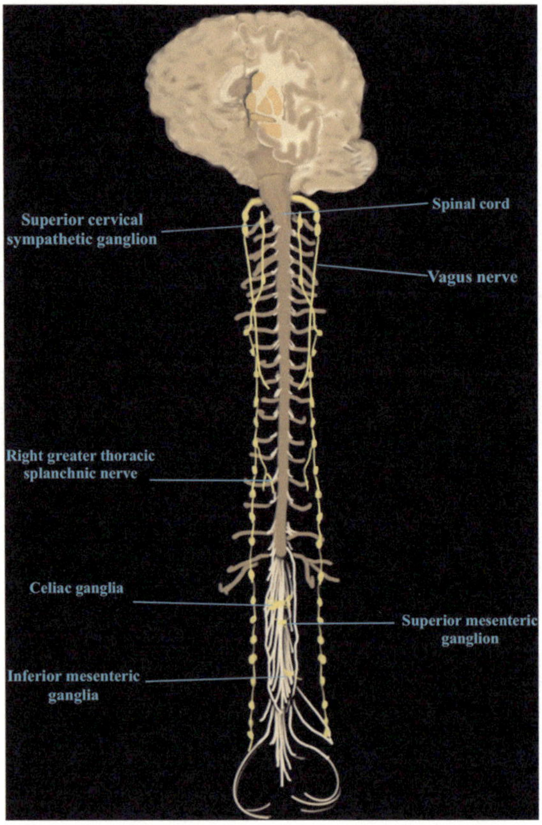

Figure 4.
Parts of the inner and outer FoK-FIP signaling transduction pathway. The FoK-FIP signaling transduction pathway.

signaling network serves a biomechanical function (e.g., bones, cartilage, tendons, and ligaments) that includes the cognitive force associated with immovable and moveable cells. The immobile population of cells develops from undifferentiated mesenchyme cells. In contrast, the mobile population of cells comprises hematopoietic stem cells, including macrophages and leukocytes. The cells of the signaling network that are critical to the EMR consciousness wavefront function are fibroblasts/fibrocytes [44], osteoblasts/osteocytes [45], chondroblasts/chondrocytes, monocytes [46], macrophages, mast cells [47]; and adipocytes (**Figures 2–6**) [49].

5. The disease: FoK-FIP D

FoK-FIP D is the maladaptive schema that occurs through the cognitive force with abnormal (i.e., hypo vs. hyper) sensitivity to the interoception of FoK-FIP. It is a transdisciplinary modeled complex disease that explains the comorbidity of mental disorders and physical conditions of animal models that emerge within the world of interoceptive cognition consciousness. The core features of FoK-FIP D include integrated perception connected with all levels of peripheral nerves, tissue modulation,

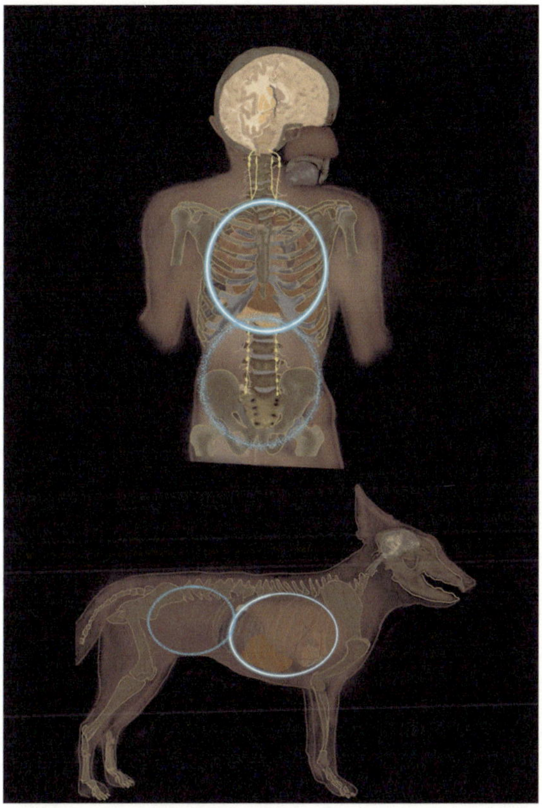

Figure 5.
In animal models, through the head, thorax, and abdominopelvic regions connected through the spinal cord and peripheral nervous tissue coupled to the EMR consciousness wavefront, there is a continuous production of the interoception of FoK-FIP. In this figure, the thorax of a human and dog model is demarcated by a solid circle, whereas a dotted circle demarcates the abdominopelvic region. The human and canine model with connected components.

and limbic system functions through the EMR consciousness wavefront spinal cord coupling. As such, the cerebral cortex's conscious intellectual functions and the brain stem's unconscious and autonomic functions connect with cognitive broadcasting activities through the cognitive force that reacts to the interoception of FoK-FIP. The core concept is that through FoK-gene expression, the cognitive force has abnormal sensitivity to the interoception of FoK-FIP. In the cellular framework represented by the animal model, the cognitive force's sensitivity is linked by the EMR consciousness wavefront coupled with the spinal cord and peripheral nervous tissue to sympathetic (originating from dorsal root ganglia) and parasympathetic (originating in the nodose ganglion of the vagus nerve or dorsal root ganglia at sacral levels) sensory neurons. There are three variations of FOK-FIP D in which FoK gene expression is abnormal due to epigenetic (i.e., some external factor influences the expression) and/or genetic factors:

5.1 Type IA

FoK gene expression is increased, and the cognitive force has increased sensitivity to the interoception of FoK-FIP. Increased myocyte contraction occurs and

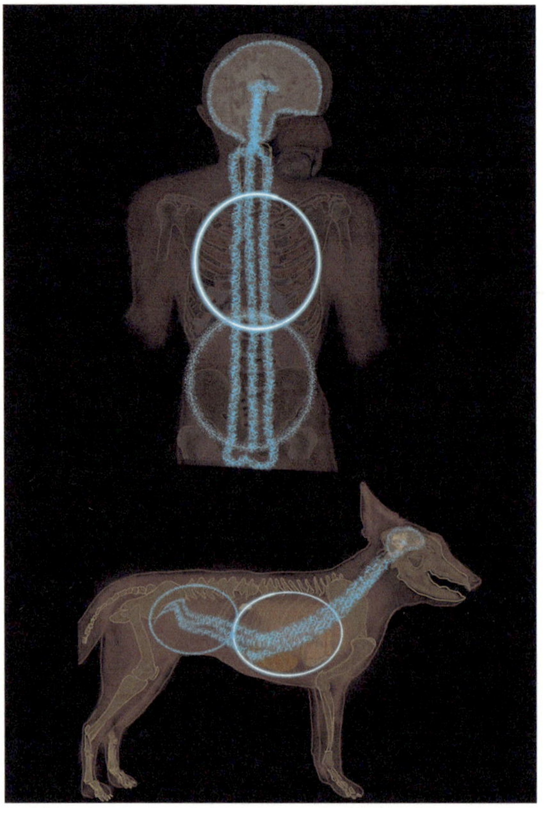

Figure 6.
The EMR consciousness wavefront coupled to the spinal cord and peripheral nervous tissue of a human and a dog model connects the head, thorax, and abdominopelvic regions. The EMR consciousness wavefront.

sympathetic nervous system hyperactivity is transmitted via the paleospinothalamic tract leading to overstimulation of the limbic system. This co-occurs with decreased gastrointestinal tract activity and signaling of the inner organs, leading to decreased afferent transmission via the vagus nerve fibers [50].

5.2 Type IB

FoK gene expression is increased, and the cognitive force has increased sensitivity to the interoception of FoK-FIP. Increased myocyte contraction occurs and sympathetic nervous system hyperactivity are transmitted via the paleospinothalamic tract with overstimulation of the limbic system.

5.3 Type IC

FoK gene expression is increased, and the cognitive force has increased sensitivity to the interoception of FoK-FIP. Decreased gastrointestinal tract activity and signaling of the inner organs lead to decreased afferent transmission via the vagus nerve fibers.

5.4 Type IIA

FoK gene expression is decreased; the cognitive force has decreased sensitivity to the interoception of FoK-FIP. Decreased myocyte contraction occurs and sympathetic nervous system hypoactivity is transmitted via the paleospinothalamic tract with under-stimulation of the limbic system. This co-occurs with increased gastrointestinal tract activity and signaling of the inner organs leading to increased afferent transmission via the vagus nerve fibers.

5.5 Type IIB

FoK gene expression is decreased; the cognitive force has decreased sensitivity to the interoception of FoK-FIP. Decreased myocyte contraction to occur and sympathetic nervous system hypoactivity is transmitted via the paleospinothalamic tract with under-stimulation of the limbic system.

5.6 Type IIC

FoK gene expression is decreased; the cognitive force has decreased sensitivity to the interoception of FoK-FIP. Increased gastrointestinal tract activity and signaling of the inner organs lead to increased afferent transmission via the vagus nerve fibers.

5.7 Type III

FoK gene mutation occurs.

6. The core concepts of the FoK-FIP MBPI

In the FoK-FIP theory, animal models that emerge in the phenomenal world of interoceptive cognition consciousness expands our understanding of genes. New physics of the cognitive force, understood through transdisciplinary modeling with the framework within a framework approach, creates the contextual bridging needed to connect quantum mechanics to medical diagnosis and intervention that includes activity-dependent plasticity. The FoK-FIP MBPI is the treatment for FoK-FIP D that includes exposure-like therapy through NMES application. NMES is the modality that perturbs the autonomic nervous system connected to the EMR consciousness wavefront coupled to the spinal cord and peripheral nervous tissue. This perturbation occurs during focused attention training and proprioception/balance exercise. In this process, the FoK-FIP MBPI, over time, facilitates durable learning through sympathetic nervous system stimulation with brain effects, including plasticity. The benefits of the intervention refer to changes in perception of the cognitive force, including those of ELF magnetic field FIP associated with adverse pain sensations. Continuous usage of the FoK-FIP MBPI aims to increase the quality of "life" (i.e., interoceptive cognition consciousness) through beneficial cognitive broadcasting effects related to the sensitivity of the cognitive force to the interoception of FoK-FIP. Higher-end cognitive broadcasting shows improvements in animal models in alertness, achievement, and mood, and reduction of aggressive outbursts. Further, the FoK-FIP MBPI techniques were formulated to provide some symptomatic relief from the downstream effects of sympathetic system upregulation, including the limbic center and the parasympathetic system being dysregulated with reduced vagal tone. Broad categories of improvement related to the FoK-FIP MBPI arise partly from alterations in neural function linked with the ability of the cognitive force to stabilize its impulsive reactivity to FoK-FIP feeling tones that underlie emotional processing.

Responses of the cognitive force can be stabilized by initiating a reaction with forethought following an impulsive reaction. This allows aspects of cognitive broadcasting to be modulated by the cognitive force, which leads to stabilizing its reactivity. It is a process envisioned through the components map model with IMs as returning to the gateway level of processing, specifically to component 4. This component allows focus on FoK-FIP feeling tones through sensory stimuli as sense impressions. In this process, subject and object are not a part of cognitive broadcasting. Instead, there is awareness of signals being broadcast cognitively without conceptual elaboration. Further, in the FoK-FIP MBPI, FoK-FIP feeling tones create an interoceptive experience vital to learning how to modulate emotional processing. When focused willingly by the cognitive force through a reaction with forethought, it is a tool that creates mental stability correlated to self-efficacy. It is suggested that practicing the FoK-FIP MBPI daily leads to the self-efficacy analogous to that needed to overcome treatment-resistant depression. The theory builds on the argument described in the literature that changes in self-efficacy drive all positive changes in treatment processes. It is predicted that, over time, the intervention will change the perception of the cognitive force of uncontrollable "distress" reactivity. In sum, the FoK-FIP MBPI is used to break up the automaticity of habitual reactions (i.e., automatic reactions followed by impulsive reactions) to FoK-FIP feeling tones by doing something different. Importantly, this intervention teaches that trying to avoid experiencing unpleasant FoK-FIP feeling tones is ineffective because the cognitive force cannot prevent them from occurring. Instead, awareness of FoK-FIP interference is expected to continue to create an intrusive "not right experience" until the cognitive force changes its relationship to unpleasant FoK-FIP feeling tones.

The FoK-FIP MBPI is a daily intervention with morning and evening formal practice sessions. The parts of the formal practice are mindfulness consisting of focused attention with or without the use of NMES, followed by NMES usage with proprioception and balance exercise derived from the physiotherapy literature [51]. Spontaneous practice is done throughout the day and represents an abbreviated form of formal practice that consists only of mindfulness practice without using NMES. In this regard, the FoK-FIP MBPI has aspects that correlate to the ancient and complex yoga practice of Indian philosophy with many different styles. Further, it also has aspects that correlate with the Buddhist psychological model (BPM) [52], mindful awareness in body-oriented therapy (MABT) [53], and inhibitory learning theory (ILT) [54]. The BPM is based on Buddhist texts called the Abhidhamma Pitaka and seeks to simplify mindfulness-based approaches such as mindfulness and attention regulation (i.e., concentration practice) that may reduce symptoms and improve well-being. It identifies mechanisms and describes what may occur during mindfulness practice. In contrast, the MABT is based on psychological and neurobiological research on understanding how interoceptive awareness facilitates regulation and an integrated sense of self, contributing to health and well-being. Further, the ILT builds on exposure-based therapy and is based on the idea that exaggerated beliefs maintain pathological fear of danger. This leads to maladaptive escape and avoidance behavior. As described by the ILT, the inhibitory learning process represents a new understanding of classical conditioning extinction that pulls away from habituation. Exposure and habituation are not prohibited, but ILT is an active learning process rather than a mechanical kind of exposure process.

The FoK-FIP MBPI consists of:

- **Mindfulness through sitting in which attention is focused**. This part of the FoK-FIP MBPI correlated to human models would be achieved through a willingness to focus on FoK-FIP feeling tones as a very specific interoceptive experience from the head, thorax, or abdominopelvic region while sitting and can be done with or without the use of NMES. Once found, the goal is to focus on it without trying to change anything. The core concept is "willingness" to practice even though it may be difficult.

- **Mindfulness through proprioception and balance exercises using NMES** This part of the FoK-FIP MBPI follows mindfulness through sitting practice (above). This part of the intervention with human models would be achieved through a willingness to focus on a very specific interoceptive experience (i.e., FoK-FIP feeling tone) from the head, thorax, or abdominopelvic region while engaged in proprioception and balance exercise using NMES. In this process, the NMES unit depolarizes motor nerves, causing muscle contractions in the abdominal or upper body regions according to a rotating schedule (**Figure** 7).

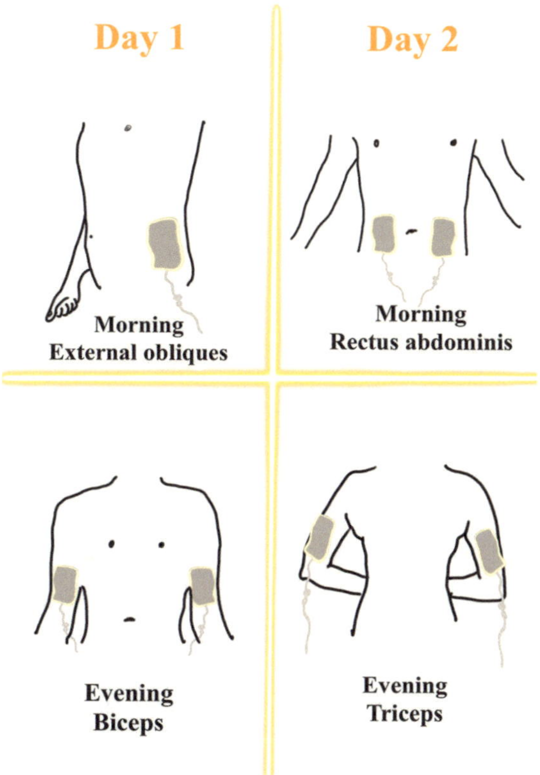

Figure 7.
This figure depicts the sites for application of the pads associated with the NMES unit applied to the skin of human models during daily use to use as part of the FoK-FIP MBPI. The human model neuromuscular electrical stimulation (NMES) schedule.

- **The spontaneous practice** in response to intrusive, unpleasant interoceptive experiences from the head, thorax, or abdominopelvic region that connects to anxious "distress," the goal is to focus on it. In this process, the willingness to practice exposure-like activity breaks up the automaticity of reacting similarly to awareness of FoK-FIP feeling tones. A hand-held "tally" counter records the momentary commitment to "challenge" rather than avoid intrusive, unpleasant interoceptive experiences.

7. The mechanistic modeling of the FoK-FIP MBPI

- ***The FoK-FIP MBPI-dependent enhancement of plasticity*** refers to the close temporal association of stimulation, proprioception, and balance exercise with focused attention on the specific events of FoK-FIP feeling tones. Engagement of neuromodulatory circuits by short trains of NMES provides a precisely timed, phasic release of neuromodulators that reinforces neural circuits activated during focused attention while engaging proprioception centers. The temporal association between NMES, proprioception/balance, and focused attention provides the specificity to target plasticity to particular neural circuits [55]. In neural circuits associated with control of the muscle groups, myocyte contraction is linked to awareness current producing ELF magnetic field FIP. The idea here is that NMES is beneficial largely by providing precise timing mediating reinforcement that supports the role of phasic activation of the cholinergic and noradrenergic systems connected to pain associated with patterns of FIP.

- **Neuromuscular electrical stimulation (NMES).** Current associated with the placement of the NMES unit's pads will follow the path of least resistance, and motor nerves depolarize, which produces muscle contractions. In this process, signals travel up sensory nerve fibers composed of axons of sensory neurons in the spinal ganglion. These axons enter the spinal cord coupled to the EMR consciousness wavefront, divide and travel short distances upward and downward one or two segments. They terminate in the outer (external) part of the spinal cord's dorsal horn. Various nerve fibers synapse in the dorsal horn, including A-alpha which are associated with proprioception (position sense), and A-beta which are related to touch. Collateral axons also penetrate the deepest layers of the dorsal horn. Additionally, the smaller-diameter fibers that transmit pain, A-delta, along with unmyelinated C fibers, synapse on two main types of neurons located in specific layers of the dorsal root of the spinal cord: The specific nociceptive neurons and non-specific neurons. The axons of the non-specific nociceptive neurons form the paleospinothalamic tract. Complex chronic pain (in contrast with acute or chronic pain) mainly stimulates the limbic system. Indirectly, the NMES enhances the benefits of the FoK-FIP MBPI by engaging the plasticity-enabling cholinergic and noradrenergic neuromodulatory systems during the sitting or standing-focused attention practice. Through the spinal cord coupled to the EMR consciousness wavefront including the extraspinal tissue of the vagus nerve, NMES stimulation drives robust, phasic neural activity in the locus coeruleus (the primary source of norepinephrine in the central nervous system). It increases norepinephrine levels in the hippocampus and cortex [56–58] and increases levels of brain-derived neurotrophic factor (BDNF, a neurotrophin strongly linked to neural plasticity) [55]. Through repeated formal practice, the FoK-FIP MBPI provides robust activation of neuromodulatory systems at specific times during training to promote substantial enhancement of plasticity, which may have benefits related to the efficacy of spontaneous practice.

- **Proprioception and balance exercise** is linked with the hypothalamus's role in stimulating or inhibiting primary bodily functions (e.g., heart rate and blood pressure, body temperature, fluid and electrolyte balance, appetite and body weight, sleep cycle and function of the gastrointestinal tract (other conditions being equal) determined by: (a). The body's posture through the total quantity of proprioceptive impulses impinging on the posterior hypothalamus per unit of time [59]. (b). Facial contraction patterns lead to afferent discharges via the hypothalamic cortical system and interact with cutaneous facial impulses in the cortex [59]. In contrast, the NMES part of the FoK-FIP MBPI builds upon the growing preclinical and clinical evidence that pairing bursts of vagus nerve stimulation with specific movements or sensory events can improve rehabilitation results [55].

- **Benefits** of the FoK-FIP MBPI are achieved through the modulation of reactions by the cognitive force occurring through the EMR consciousness wavefront coupled to the spinal cord and peripheral nervous tissue. These effects correlate with the modulation of neural circuit signaling, including that of the paleospinothalamic tract and a peripheral nervous tissue pathway of the nodose ganglion, with information traveling to the brain stem via the vagus nerve. The automatic and impulsive reactions of the cognitive force correlate with afferent activation of the paleospinothalamic tract and excitatory sympathetic input to the brain. In contrast, the impulsive reaction followed by the reaction with forethought by the cognitive force correlates with a calming parasympathetic outflow through efferent activation. The benefits through the reactions of the cognitive force linked with the activation of the limbic and proprioception centers and the stimulation of the vagus nerve at the cervical level have beneficial effects on the broadcasting for "life" (i.e., interoceptive cognition consciousness).

8. Infrared thermal imaging to test aspects of the FoK-FIP theory

The reaction of the sensitive cognitive force to the interoception of FoK-FIP is the mechanism modulating the cognitive broadcasting of signals occurring through the EMR consciousness wavefront coupled to the spinal cord and peripheral nervous tissue. In the testing environment, a thermal camera receives infrared radiation emitted from the canine participants' cervical, thoracic and lumbar regions, and the system's technology produces radiometric video. Infrared thermal imaging (IRT) is a non-ionizing, non-invasive technique to evaluate the comfort levels of animals (e.g., human and non-human). Through electromagnetic waves, an objective relationship exists between:

- Parts of EMR consciousness wavefront cognitively broadcast by the sensitive cognitive force with "distress."

- Animal models' physiopathological alterations through microvascular changes [60] associated with autonomic arousal during normal vigilance versus hypervigilance (shown by hyperactivity, impulsivity, and inattention).

- Thermal windows show aspects of chunking and stimulus organization of pixels by the cognitive force that produces components of interoceptive cognition consciousness (envisioned through the components map model with IMs). In this process, a radiometric thermal imaging system (i.e., Teletherm TIGER-4 infrared thermal imager) detects thermal radiation as a particular property of the EMR consciousness wavefront.

9. Conclusions

This chapter has introduced the FoK-FIP MBPI and has shown how the FoK-FIP theory contributes broadly to the scientific literature, including theoretical and classical theory, empirical research, biology, and medical diagnosis, and intervention.

Acknowledgements

The author would like to thank Graham J. Rockley for his support, including the technical that expedited the learning of the Teletherm Tiger 4 Cub Infrared Thermal Imaging System.

Conflict of interest

The author declares no conflict of interest.

Author details

Holly Pollard-Wright
Institute of Electrical and Electronics Engineers (IEEE), National Coalition of Independent Scholars (NCIS), United States of America

*Address all correspondence to: holly.pollard-wright@ncis.org

References

[1] Pollard-Wright H. Feelings of knowing—fundamental interoceptive patterns (FoK-FIP): A magnetic monopole-like "pure mental" process fundamental to subjective feelings and self-awareness. Communicative & Integrative Biology. 2022;**15**(1):1-54. DOI: 10.1080/19420889.2021.2023280

[2] Pollard-Wright H. A unifying theory of physics and biological information through consciousness. Communicative & Integrative Biology. 2021;**14**(1):78-110. DOI: 10.1080/19420889.2021.1907910

[3] Pollard-Wright H. Interoception the foundation for: Mind's sensing of "self," physiological responses, cognitive discrimination and dysregulation. Communicative & Integrative Biology. 2020;**13**(1):198-213. DOI: 10.1080/19420889.2020.1846922

[4] Pollard-Wright H. Electrochemical energy, primordial feelings and feelings of knowing (FOK): Mindfulness-based intervention for interoceptive experience related to phobic and anxiety disorders. Medical Hypotheses. 2020;**144**:109909. DOI: 10.1016/j.mehy.2020.109909

[5] Pollard-Wright H. The feelings of knowing—fundamental interoceptive patterns (FoK-FIP) system: Connecting consciousness to physics. Communicative & Integrative Biology. 27 Sep 2023;**16**(1):2260682. DOI: 10.1080/19420889.2023.2260682. PMID: 37779822; PMCID: PMC10538454

[6] Horgan J. Troublemaker Lee Smolin Says Physics–And its Laws–Must Evolve. New York, NY: Springer Nature America, Inc. (Scientific American); 2015. Available from: https://blogs.scientificamerican.com/cross-check/troublemaker-lee-smolin-says-physics-8211-and-its-laws-8211-must-evolve/

[7] Koriat A. The feeling of knowing: Some metatheoretical implications for consciousness and control. Consciousness and Cognition. 2000;**9**(2):149-171. DOI: 10.1006/ccog.2000.0433

[8] Davies P. Does new physics lurk inside living matter? Physics Today. 2020;**73**(8):34-40. DOI: 10.1063/PT.3.4546

[9] Ogata N. Separation anxiety in dogs: What progress has been made in our understanding of the most common behavioral problems in dogs? Journal of Veterinary Behavior. 2016;**16**:28-35. DOI: 10.1016/j.jveb.2016.02.005

[10] Rab-Gsal-Zla-Ba, Mkhyen-Brtse D-M, Ricard M, Kurz V. The Collected Works of Dilgo Khyentse. Boulder, Colorado, USA: Shambhala Publications, Inc; 2010

[11] Wilczek F. A beautiful question: finding nature's deep design. New York: Penguin Books; 2016

[12] Liboff AR. Toward an electromagnetic paradigm for biology and medicine. The Journal of Alternative and Complementary Medicine. 2004;**10**(1):41-47. DOI: 10.1089/107555304322848940

[13] Schrödinger E. What Is Life? The Physical Aspect of the Living Cell. Cambridge, United Kingdom: Cambridge University Press; 1944

[14] Roberts D. Writer's Web: Reasoning: General Inferential Errors. VA, USA:

University of Richmond; 2010. Available from: http://writing2.richmond.edu/writing/wweb/reason2a.html

[15] Adolphs R. The biology of fear. Current Biology. 2013;**23**(2):R79-R93. DOI: 10.1016/j.cub.2012.11.055

[16] Baars B. Consciousness. Scholarpedia. 2015;**10**(8):2207. DOI: 10.4249/scholarpedia.2207

[17] Forrester JW. World Dynamics. Lawrence, Kansas: Wright-Allen Press, Cop; 1971

[18] Shi Z, Wang X, Yue J. Cognitive cycle in mind model CAM. International Journal of Intelligence Science. 2011;**1**(2):25-34. DOI: 10.4236/ijis.2011.12004

[19] Cohen D. Magnetic fields of the human body. Physics Today. 1975;**28**(8):34-43. DOI: 10.1063/1.3069110

[20] Gmbh V, Verlag V. Essential Facts of Physical Medicine, Rehabilitation and Sports Medicine in Companion Animals. Babenhausen, Germany: Babenhausen Vbs Vetverlag; 2019

[21] Celano CM, Daunis DJ, Lokko HN, Campbell KA, Huffman JC. Anxiety disorders and cardiovascular disease. Current Psychiatry Reports. 2016;**18**(11):101. DOI: 10.1007/s11920-016-0739-5

[22] Sardinha A, Freire RC, Zin DRWA, Nardi AE. Respiratory manifestations of panic disorder: Causes, consequences and therapeutic implications. Jornal Brasileiro de Pneumologia. 2009;**35**(7):698-708. DOI: 10.1590/s1806-37132009000700012

[23] Zhang K, Sakamoto A, Chang L, Qu Y, Wang S, Pu Y, et al. Splenic NKG2D confers resilience versus susceptibility in mice after chronic social defeat stress: Beneficial effects of (R)-ketamine. European Archives of Psychiatry and Clinical Neuroscience. 2019;**271**(3):447-456. DOI: 10.1007/s00406-019-01092-z

[24] Wei Y, Wang T, Liao L, Fan X, Chang L, Hashimoto K. Brain-spleen axis in health and diseases: A review and future perspective. Brain Research Bulletin. 2022;**182**:130-140. DOI: 10.1016/j.brainresbull.2022.02.008

[25] Choi JM, Chung GE, Kang SJ, Kwak M-S, Yang JI, Park B, et al. Association between anxiety and depression and nonalcoholic fatty liver disease. Frontiers in Medicine. 2021;**7**:585618. DOI: 10.3389/fmed.2020.585618

[26] Dunbar EK, Saloman JL, Phillips AE, Whitcomb DC. Severe pain in chronic pancreatitis patients: Considering mental health and associated genetic factors. Journal of Pain Research. 2021;**14**:773-784. DOI: 10.2147/JPR.S274276

[27] Lkhagvasuren B, Mee-inta O, Zhao Z-W, Hiramoto T, Boldbaatar D, Kuo Y-M. Pancreas-brain crosstalk. Frontiers in Neuroanatomy. 2021;**15**:691777. DOI: 10.3389/fnana.2021.691777

[28] Gutkowska J, Jankowski M, Lambert C, Mukaddam-Daher S, Zingg HH, McCann SM. Oxytocin releases atrial natriuretic peptide by combining with oxytocin receptors in the heart. Proceedings of the National Academy of Sciences. 1997;**94**(21):11704-11709. DOI: 10.1073/pnas.94.21.11704

[29] Jankowski M, Broderick TL, Gutkowska J. The role of oxytocin in cardiovascular protection. Frontiers in Psychology. 2020;**11**:2139. DOI: 10.3389/fpsyg.2020.02139

[30] Jankowski M, Hajjar F, Kawas SA, Mukaddam-Daher S, Hoffman G, McCann SM, et al. Rat heart: A site of oxytocin production and action. Proceedings. National Academy of Sciences. United States of America. 1998; **95**:14558-14563. DOI: 10.1073/pnas.95.24.14558

[31] Japundzic-Zigon N. Vasopressin and oxytocin in control of the cardiovascular system. Current Neuropharmacology. 2013;**11**:218-230. DOI: 10.2174/1570159x11311020008

[32] Kirsch P. Oxytocin in the socioemotional brain: Implications for psychiatric disorders. Dialogues in Clinical Neuroscience. 2015;**17**(4):463-476

[33] Thibonnier M, Conarty DM, Preston JA, Plesnicher CL, Dweik RA, Erzurum SC. Human vascular endothelial cells express oxytocin receptors. Endocrinology. 1999;**140**:1301-1309. DOI: 10.1210/endo.140.3.6546

[34] Cattaneo MG, Lucci G, Vicentini LM. Oxytocin stimulates in vitro angiogenesis via a Pyk-2/Src-dependent mechanism. Experimental Cell Research. 2009;**315**:3210-3219. DOI: 10.1016/j.yexcr.2009.06.022

[35] Sali AW, Anderson BA, Courtney SM. Information processing biases in the brain: Implications for decision-making and self-governance. Neuroethics. 2016;**11**(3):259-271. DOI: 10.1007/s12152-016-9251-1

[36] Philippi CL, Feinstein JS, Khalsa SS, Damasio A, Tranel D, Landini G, et al. Preserved self-awareness following extensive bilateral brain damage to the insula, anterior cingulate, and medial prefrontal cortices. PLoS One. 2012;7(8):e38413. DOI: 10.1371/journal.pone.0038413

[37] Wolff M, Vann SD. The cognitive thalamus as a gateway to mental representations. The Journal of Neuroscience. 2018;**39**(1):3-14. DOI: 10.1523/jneurosci.0479-18.2018

[38] Jobson DD, Hase Y, Clarkson AN, Kalaria RN. The role of the medial prefrontal cortex in cognition, ageing and dementia. Brain Communications. 2021;**3**(3):fcab125. DOI: 10.1093/braincomms/fcab125

[39] Báez-Mendoza R, Schultz W. The role of the striatum in social behavior. Frontiers in Neuroscience. 2013;7:233. DOI: 10.3389/fnins.2013.00233

[40] Schmahmann JD. The cerebellum and cognition. Neuroscience Letters. 2019;**688**:62-75. DOI: 10.1016/j.neulet.2018.07.005

[41] Madl T, Baars BJ, Franklin S. The timing of the cognitive cycle. PLoS One. 2011;**6**(4):e14803. DOI: 10.1371/journal.pone.0014803

[42] Milardi D, Bramanti P, Milazzo C, Finocchio G, Arrigo A, Santoro G, et al. Cortical and subcortical connections of the human claustrum revealed In vivo by constrained spherical deconvolution tractography. Cerebral Cortex. 2013; **25**(2):406-414. DOI: 10.1093/cercor/bht231

[43] Benarroch EE. What is the role of the claustrum in cortical function and neurologic disease? Neurology. 2021; **96**(3):110-113. DOI: 10.1212/WNL.0000000000011280

[44] Olesen MA, Villavicencio-Tejo F, Quintanilla RA. The use of fibroblasts as a valuable strategy for studying mitochondrial impairment in

neurological disorders. Translational Neurodegeneration. 2022;**11**:36. DOI: 10.1186/s40035-022-00308-y

[45] Delgado-Calle JM, Bellido T. The osteocyte as a signaling cell. Physiological Reviews. 2021;**102**: 379-410. DOI: 10.1152/physrev. 00043.2020

[46] Wohleb ES, McKim DB, Sheridan JF, Godbout JP. Monocyte trafficking to the brain with stress and inflammation: A novel axis of immune-to-brain communication that influences mood and behavior. Frontiers in Neuroscience. 2015;**8**:447. DOI: 10.3389/ fnins.2014.00447

[47] Nautiyal KM, Ribeiro AC, Pfaff DW, Silver R. Brain mast cells link the immune system to anxiety-like behavior. Proceedings of the National Academy of Sciences. 2008;**105**(46):18053-18057. DOI: 10.1073/pnas.0809479105

[48] Netter FH, Dalley AF. Atlas of Human Anatomy. Teterboro: Icon Learning Systems; 2003

[49] Eichwald T, Talbot S. Neuro-immunity controls obesity-induced pain. Frontiers in Human Neuroscience. 2020; **14**:181. DOI: 10.3389/fnhum.2020.00181

[50] Breit S, Kupferberg A, Rogler G, Hasler G. Vagus nerve as modulator of the brain–gut Axis in psychiatric and inflammatory disorders. Frontiers in Psychiatry. 2018;**9**:44. DOI: 10.3389/ fpsyt.2018.00044

[51] Millis DL, Levine D. Canine Rehabilitation and Physical Therapy. 2nd ed. Philadelphia, USA: Elsevier Science Publishers; 2014, Cop

[52] Grabovac AD, Lau MA, Willett BR. Mechanisms of mindfulness: A Buddhist psychological model. Mindfulness. 2011; **2**(3):154-166

[53] Price CJ, Hooven C. Interoceptive awareness skills for emotion regulation: Theory and approach of mindful awareness in body-oriented therapy (MABT). Frontiers in Psychology. 2018; **9**:798. DOI: 10.3389/fpsyg.2018.00798

[54] Jacoby RJ, Abramowitz JS. Inhibitory learning approaches to exposure therapy: A critical review and translation to obsessive-compulsive disorder. Clinical Psychology Review. 2016;**49**:28-40. DOI: 10.1016/j.cpr.2016.07.001

[55] Engineer CT, Hays SA, Kilgard MP. Vagus nerve stimulation as a potential adjuvant to behavioral therapy for autism and other neurodevelopmental disorders. Journal of Neurodevelopmental Disorders. 2017;**9**(1):20. DOI: 10.1186/s11689-017-9203-z

[56] Hassert DL, Miyashita T, Williams CL. The effects of peripheral vagal nerve stimulation at a memory-modulating intensity on norepinephrine output in the basolateral amygdala. Behavioral Neuroscience. 2004;**118**: 79-88

[57] Roosevelt RW, Smith DC, Clough RW, Jensen RA, Browning RA. Increased extracellular concentrations of norepinephrine in cortex and hippocampus following vagus nerve stimulation in the rat. Brain Research. 2006;**1119**:124-132

[58] Follesa P, Biggio F, Gorini G, Caria S, Talani G, Dazzi L, et al. Vagus nerve stimulation increases norepinephrine concentration and the gene expression of BDNF and bFGF in the rat brain. Brain Research. 2007;**1179**:28-34

[59] Gellhorn E. Motion and emotion: The role of proprioception in the physiology and pathology of the

emotions. Psychological Review. 1964; **71**(6):457-472. DOI: 10.1037/h0039834

[60] Mota-Rojas D, Pereira AMF, Wang D, Martínez-Burnes J, Ghezzi M, Hernández-Avalos I, et al. Clinical applications and factors involved in validating thermal windows used in infrared thermography in cattle and river Buffalo to assess health and productivity. Animals (Basel). 2021; **11**(8):2247. DOI: 10.3390/ani11082247